A FIRESIDE BOOK
Published by
Simon & Schuster

NEW YORK   LONDON   TORONTO   SYDNEY   TOKYO   SINGAPORE

THE

FAST-
FOOD
DIET

QUICK AND HEALTHY EATING

AT HOME AND ON THE GO

MARY DONKERSLOOT, R.D.

FIRESIDE
Simon & Schuster Building
Rockefeller Center
1230 Avenue of the Americas
New York, New York   10020

First Fireside Edition 1992

FIRESIDE and colophon are registered trademarks
of Simon & Schuster Inc.

Designed by Liney Li
Manufactured in the United States of America

10 9 8 7 6 5 4 3 2 1
10 9 8 7 6 5 4   Pbk.

Library of Congress Cataloging in Publication Data

Donkersloot, Mary, date.
    The fast-food diet : quick and healthy eating at home and on the
go / by Mary Donkersloot.
        p.   cm.
    Includes index.
    1. Reducing diets.   2. Convenience foods.   I. Title.
RM222.2.D665   1991
613.2'5—dc20   90-47143
                                                                CIP

ISBN 0-671-69391-3
ISBN: 0-671-75446-7 Pbk.

TO MOM,
for nourishing
my body and soul
over the years.

ACKNOWLEDGMENTS

THIS book did not come from me alone. I would like to thank my family, friends, and colleagues whose invaluable support made this book possible.

First, I must thank my agent, David Rorvik, Proteus, Inc., for his expert collaboration in our mutual endeavor. In addition, I thank Siri Moore for her assistance in research, analysis, and long hours at her computer rating foods from 1 to 10. I also thank Lisa Carlson, M.S., R.D., for her work in editing the book. And, of course I thank Bob Bender, my editor at Simon and Schuster for his support.

To the following individuals who contributed their professional expertise, I am deeply indebted: Barbara Grasse, R.D., D.B.E.; Susan Algert, M.S., R.D.; Joan Rupp, M.S., R.D.; Robert Antonacci, M.S., Exercise Physiology; Cheryl Rock, M.S., R.D.; Jim Moore, Computer Advisor; Steven Van Camp, M.D.; and Diane Hastings.

I thank the hundreds of individuals who have worked with me to learn fast and healthy ways of eating that support their personal health and weight goals.

And, of course, I thank my parents, Ed and Alma Donkersloot, for their love and staunch belief in me. I thank my friends Mar Birgisson and Jennifer Luce for being there daily. To my friends, Bill Ballance, Ruth Bergstrom, Betty Byrnes, Dennis Clark, Don Fells, Terry Graves, Raul Guerrero, Jackie Horner, Robert Jaye, Bok and Suzy Lee, Sheldon Lerner, Rocky Nitchels, Randy Robbins, Terry and Joey Sapp, Peter Snell, Deborah St. George, Dennis Stubblefield, Scott Wade, and Frankie Wright, thank you all for tasting, reading, and rereading as well as for your love, distraction, and encouragement.

CONTENTS

PART 1

FAST FOODS CAN BE *HEALTHY* FOODS

CHAPTER · 1

WHAT THE FAST-FOOD DIET CAN DO FOR *YOU*

A *HEALTHY* DIET FOR PEOPLE IN A *HURRY*

How many times have you heard someone lament, "I *would* eat a healthy diet if only I had the *time*." This familiar complaint is behind the growth of such fast-food franchises as McDonald's, Burger King, Wendy's and Roy Rogers. "Fast food" includes take-out deli foods, frozen food, and other convenience foods. These foods come from supermarkets, delis, bakeries, pizza parlors, and, of course, the quick-service restaurants that helped coin the term, "fast food." Fast food means fast shopping, fast cooking, and fast eating—foods that can be purchased and eaten quickly. By these criteria, apples are fast foods.

We all depend on fast foods from time to time—foods that are either already prepared or can be prepared in ten to twenty minutes. According to a survey on dining time by Food Marketing Institute and *Better Homes and Gardens* magazine, only 34 percent of quick dinners are homemade, while 32 percent are frozen and 20 percent supermarket take-out. In this survey, quick-dinner food preferences, listed in order, were burgers, pasta, sandwiches, soup, poultry, pizza, hot dogs, and lastly, salad.

Unfortunately, many of these "fast foods" that have become mainstays in the American diet are fairly high in calories, sodium, and fat, particularly saturated fat, and lacking in useful fiber, vitamins, minerals, and other essential micronutrients. This type of diet contributes enormously to obesity, and has been a risk factor for heart disease and cancer.

But there is good news for busy people who have to eat in a hurry, and that good news is what this book is all about. It delivers a *nutritionally sound* fast-food diet, one that can actually help you lose weight, give you more energy, help make you feel better about yourself and make you healthier. And the Fast-Food Diet does this *without* requiring that you alter your lifestyle or spend more time in the kitchen than you currently do! The diet not only helps you lose weight—but helps you keep it off permanently.

A LIFESAVING GUIDE THROUGH THE FAST-FOOD JUNGLE

The Fast-Food Diet safely guides the harried and the hurried through today's fast-food jungle. The diet provides detailed guidelines, analyses, ratings, and recommendations related to all manner of fast foods from supermarkets, delis, frozen foods, snacks, desserts of all kinds, and, of course, the offerings of all the major fast-food chains. It tells you which food items are the best, which are the worst, and everything in between.

Fortunately, we're beginning to see signs of a "kinder, gentler" jungle. Even the franchisers are beginning to offer healthier fare. This book will help you find the best of the new fast foods and avoid the worst of the old. If you follow the Fast-Food Diet, you can reduce your intake of fat from around 40 percent to less than 30 percent, with less than 10 percent saturated fat. You can decide how far you want to go. Whatever you choose, you will still get to eat delicious food that either comes already prepared or which takes no more than twenty minutes to prepare.

In addition to lowering your fat and cholesterol intake, you'll also be reducing your sodium consumption and increasing your fiber intake when you follow the Fast-Food Diet. This program also helps you get optimal amounts of protein and complex carbohydrates, along with vitamins, minerals, and other micronutrients.

You'll find the rating system simple and easy to use. All of the fast foods are rated on a scale of 1 to 10. The higher the rating the better the choice. Which is healthier: a Big Mac or a Quarter Pounder with cheese, an Egg McMuffin or pancakes? The answers will often surprise you, even as they instruct you (see Chapter 8).

You'll find individual chapters on fast-food breakfasts, lunches, and dinners. These will provide you with easy-to-implement guidelines aimed at making main meals fast and healthy, whether you're eating at home; brown bagging on the job; or eating out at a restaurant, a fast-food franchise, or taking out from a deli or a supermarket. These chapters are packed with how-to tips to save you time and provide you with healthy fare that is not only fast but exciting and varied. These are augmented by additional chapters on snacks, desserts, and beverages. The fast-food snacking system will not only keep you satisfied, it will also help you prevent weight gain and keep you fit. Snack bars, cookies, nuts and seeds, fruit and fruit snacks, crackers and chips, vegetable snacks, desserts, and beverages all get rated.

THE FAST-FOOD WEIGHT-LOSS PLAN

Eating "fast" has usually meant eating "fat," but the Fast-Food Diet changes that. Most of the people who consult me at my company, Personal Nutrition Management, are very active people; many of them were overweight when they first came to me. Most are now right where they want to be in the weight department—and they got there without having to change their lifestyles. They're all as active as ever, but now they are also more productive than ever thanks to being leaner and fitter. The Fast-Food Weight-Loss Plan provides selections at four different caloric levels. Menu plans for twenty-one days are also provided, as is an exercise program you can actually stick with.

COMPREHEN-SIVE RATINGS

In addition to the many ratings you'll find in the meal chapters, the final chapter in Part I provides extensive ratings of all the major franchise foods currently available. You'll find ratings for the offerings of McDonald's, Burger King, Wendy's, Hardee's, Pizza Hut, Taco Bell, Kentucky Fried Chicken, Domino's, Dairy Queen, Carl's Jr., Jack in the Box, Arthur Treacher's, Arby's, Long John Silver's, and Roy Rogers.

You'll also find the fast-food rating of familiar frozen foods, including Healthy Choice, Right Choice, Stouffer's Lean Cuisine, Light and Elegant, Banquet, Pillsbury, Budget Gourmet, Weight Watchers, Armour Dinner Classics, Benihana Oriental Lites, Le Menu, and Mrs. Paul's.

THE FAST-FOOD RECIPES

Part II of this book consists of more than a hundred fast-food recipes—fast-food meals you can prepare for consumption on the road, at home, or in the office—in twenty minutes or less!

These include breakfasts, brown-bag specials, salads and salad dressings, soups, main dishes, party snacks, and desserts. These tasty swifties have proved enormously popular with my clients. So popular, in fact, that I put together a "Fast Food at Home" recipe box for my clients. They spread the word, and soon publications such as *Glamour* and *American Health* were commenting favorably on my little red box of recipes. In a matter of weeks, I was inundated with thousands of orders. That's when I decided I'd better write a book—to explain the *healthy* fast-food philosophy and expand on the fast-food recipes.

This is that book: your guide to living fast, eating well, and feeling better.

CHAPTER · 2

THE FAST-FOOD RATING SYSTEM

People continually ask me for nutritional advice about specific foods. "How bad is it if I eat a pizza once a week? Or a Big Mac and fries? What if I only eat bacon and eggs a few times a month? Can't I occasionally replace a real dinner with a margarita and chips? How do chocolate chip cookies and ice cream fit in?" Answers such as, "It's terrible, don't eat it," or "Go ahead, it's not that bad," make me cringe, both for their imprecision and their cop-out quality.

"TELL ME, ON A SCALE OF 1 TO 10 . . ."

To help provide *real* answers, I have developed the Fast-Food Rating Scale, a very simple but scientific system that rates foods from 1 to 10. The initial inspiration for the creation of the rating scale was the exasperated response I got one day from a client, while trying to explain to her, in complex terms, why her beloved Bacon, Egg, and Cheese Croissan'wich (a Burger King offering) is a fast-food peril.

"Oh," she moaned, "can't you just tell me on a scale of 1 to 10 how it stacks up with other foods?"

"About a one," I said. This made my point—and it set me to thinking. If I *really* could devise such a scale, based on sound nutritional considerations, it would certainly make life easier for all of my clients—and for consumers everywhere. After considerable further study, I found that I was, in fact, able to construct such a scale. One of the first things I did after completing it, was to call the client mentioned above to tell her I'd made a mistake. Her favorite food is actually a 2, not a 1.

The scale is based on factors identified in the 1988 "U.S. Surgeon General's Report on Health and Nutrition." The scale takes into account total fat, saturated fat, cholesterol, salt, sugar, fiber, vitamins, and minerals. The best rating is 10, the worst is 1.

The Fast-Food Rating Scale shows people the whole picture, with *one* number. How much total fat, saturated fat, and cholesterol are in the food? Because these factors have the most significant bearing on health issues facing most Americans, they account for more points on the scale. Fiber also affects the quality of the diet, and I haven't forgotten salt either, although I have been a bit more liberal with it than some authorities have, primarily because the existing data related to the effects of salt on health are not as strong. The scale reflects today's concerns over a diet of excess fat and cholesterol, rather than a diet deficient in vitamins and minerals. (See Appendix A for further details about the rating system.)

As you look at the rating charts in subsequent chapters, **note that the factors that most detract from a food's nutritional value are boldfaced.** This will help you if you have a particular problem. For example, if you have had a heart attack or have high blood cholesterol, your doctor or dietitian will suggest that you alter your diet. You can zero in on cholesterol and saturated-fat content of foods in the ratings.

You may notice that there is no rating for calories. This is because individual need varies greatly, depending on body/frame size, sex, and activity level. However, you can frequently rely on a food's fat content as a predictor of its calorie content. Generally speaking, the more fat, the more calories, while the reverse is also true: less fat, fewer calories. Fat delivers more than twice the calories ounce for ounce, as carbohydrates or protein do.

Calculations have been based on a *per serving* and *per meal* basis rather than per ounce or per specific volume, because I want you to relate the score to the portion that you actually eat. If you eat very large or very small servings, then make the adjustment between the figures I give and the portion size you eat.

The nutrient content of foods has been derived from data supplied by food companies, fast-food restaurants; packaging labels; USDA *Handbook 8*; and *Bowes and Church's Food Values of Portions Commonly Used*, 15th edition, 1989.

Many charts specify brand names, fast-food chains, and specific franchise foods. No endorsement of any product or brand name is implied or intended.

DIETARY OBJECTIVES OF THE FAST-FOOD RATING SCALE

Lower the Fat in Your Diet

Less fat means a decreased risk of coronary artery disease and fewer calories. Most Americans get about 37 to 40 percent of their calories from fat. In fact, new research from Jean-Pierre Flatt, Ph.D. of the University of Massachusetts Medical School, indicates that calories from dietary fat (such as butter), are *more* fattening than calories from carbohydrates (such as bread), because fat requires less energy to be processed within the body. The American Heart Association and the National Cholesterol Education Program (NCEP) recommend reducing total fat intake to 30 percent of calories or less, and reducing saturated fat to 10 percent. If you know how many calories you need, you can determine the 30 percent into fat grams. The chart below can help.

Suggested Fat Intake ☛

DAILY CALORIE LEVEL	MAXIMUM GRAMS OF TOTAL FAT	MAXIMUM GRAMS OF SATURATED FAT
1000	33	11
1200	40	13
1400	47	16
1600	53	18
1800	60	20
2000	67	22
2200	73	24
2400	80	27
2600	87	29
2800	93	31
3000	100	33

Daily fat intake is determined by the following formula:
Total fat
Total calories × 30% = daily calories from fat ÷ 9 = _____ grams total fat
(Example: 1800 calories × .30 = 540 ÷ 9 = 60 grams)
Saturated fat
Total calories × 10% = daily calories from saturated fat ÷ 9 = _____ grams saturated fat
(Example: 1800 calories × .10 = 180 ÷ 9 = 20 grams)

Check labels to see how many grams of fat are in the foods you eat. Use lean meats, and limit added fats from toppings such as butter, margarine, or mayonnaise, and choose new low-fat or no-fat desserts. Use low-fat or nonfat dairy products to replace excessive saturated fat, cholesterol, and calories from butterfat. Refer to Appendix B for fat grams in common foods. This will help you stay within the less-than-30-percent total fat goal. By selecting fast foods with the recommended scores—specified later in this chapter—you'll automatically head toward this goal.

Eat Less Saturated Fat

Reduce your fat intake from saturated sources, such as meat and dairy products, and replace it with polyunsaturated and monounsaturated fat, usually derived from vegetable sources. The Fast-Food Diet helps you *automatically* reduce saturated fat intake to less than 10 percent of total daily calories, and *that* is one of the most important things you can do for your body. Studies show that saturated fats promote the most dangerous forms of cholesterol buildup and have two times more cholesterol-raising potential than cholesterol itself.

Limit Cholesterol

Cholesterol in the Fast-Food Diet is limited to less than 300 milligrams per day. Here's an example of what provides 300 milligrams: 2 ounces of animal protein (meat or cheese) at lunch and 3 to 4 ounces at dinner, with low-fat milk, an oil-based salad dressing, and two visible eggs *per week*. (This was adjusted in 1989 when cholesterol content of eggs was found to be *213* milligrams instead of *250*.) You'll also find the amount of cholesterol listed in the fast-food charts that appear throughout this book.

Have Adequate, but Not Excessive Protein

Protein builds and repairs muscle tissue. Obviously, we need protein, but most of us get too much. Research has shown that the average American eats more than twice the protein required, even with a heavy exercise schedule. Consequently, our Fast-Food Rating Scale gives no direct rating for protein. Instead, the protein content is reflected to a degree in the fat evaluation, since many foods high in protein are also high in fat. We want to focus on protein sources that are *not* high in saturated fat or total fat.

Eat small portions of *low-fat* protein foods, 3 to 4 ounces, once or twice per day, up to 7 or 8 ounces *total* daily. This includes lean meats trimmed of visible fat, skinless poultry, and legumes (dried peas, beans, and lentils), all cooked with minimal or no fat. Low-fat dairy products—cheese and milk—are also included in the Fast-Food Diet. Fish and shellfish are recommended at least two to three times a week to provide valuable fish oils. You'll get 12 to 18 percent of your total calories from protein on the Fast-Food Diet.

Eat More Complex Carbohydrates

Fast living calls for *complex* carbohydrates—pasta, potatoes, rice, vegetables, whole-grain breads and cereals, for 55 to 65 percent of total calories. Complex carbohydrates are the most efficient source of energy—the kind the muscles can use most readily. They generally provide a low-fat source of protein when added fats are limited. Carbohydrates are more easily broken down than fats or protein (primarily because of their ideal ratio of carbon-hydrogen-oxygen), so they are used when the body needs an immediate burst of energy. The body's fat is used for energy only after twenty to thirty minutes of deliberate exercise at an elevated heart rate. People who skip carbohydrates are likely to feel tired during the day and may not have much energy; they certainly won't feel like exercising. But don't go overboard, either. The most common food-related cause of low energy level is *too much* food—whether it is carbohydrate, protein, or fat. The advice to increase carbohydrate comes from our knowledge that the typical American diet is relatively too high in fat.

Limit, but do not exclude, sugar, a *simple* carbohydrate, whether it comes from honey, table sugar, or corn sweetener. Sugar is typically found in our diets from candy, cookies, pie, cake, ice cream, jams, jellies, syrups, and soft drinks. Sugar should provide less than 10 percent of total calories, within the 55 percent carbohydrate goal.

Increase Fiber Intake

Include in each day's menu five to six servings of foods high in fiber, both the kind of soluble fiber that helps the body eliminate cholesterol and insoluble fiber that may help prevent constipation and colon cancer. To achieve the goal of 30 grams per day, such foods as oatmeal, oat bran, rice bran, psyllium, apples, pears, citrus fruits, dried peas, beans, and lentils, as well as many vegetables should be eaten. (See Appendix C for more information on fiber in foods.)

Limit Sodium

Sodium is limited to a total of 2,400 milligrams a day from all sources, in accordance with National Academy of Science recommendations. This massive study, completed in 1988, with 10,097 subjects by 52 centers in 32 countries around the world found a relatively weak link between sodium and blood pressure. Although a diet high in sodium is one of the risk factors for developing high blood pressure, the Intersalt Study indicates that only one third of people without high blood pressure are considered "salt sensitive" and need to be careful about their sodium intake, and half of those people *with* high blood pressure are salt sensitive. Unfortunately, we do not know who is and who is not salt sensitive. So a moderate level of caution is advised. Less sodium comes naturally with less-processed foods—fresh fruits, vegetables, whole grains, and meats are all safe. (See Appendix D for information on sodium content of food.)

Get an Adequate Amount of Vitamins and Minerals

The Fast-Food Diet promotes a better balance of foods, but some of you may still not get enough vitamins and minerals. For those who limit calories, travel frequently, or tend to skip one of the food groups, a supplement containing 100 percent of the RDAs* of vitamins and minerals is a good insurance policy. Foods that are skipped are often vegetables and fruits. According to a study by the California Department of Health Services in 1990, even when produce is most available, 20 percent of the population eat no fruit, and 27 percent eat no vegetables or salad. The "Strive for Five" program encourages people to eat at least five servings a day of fruit and vegetables as part of a low-fat, high-fiber diet for good health and to reduce cancer risk. Refined grains are enriched to provide as many of certain nutrients as whole grains, but the refined grains still may not have the fiber, among other things. Supplements can help, but remember that even a vitamin pill won't make up for a diet with too much fat and cholesterol and not enough fiber.

Note that it is more difficult to meet the RDA for some nutrients than others. Vitamin C is relatively easy to meet with just one serving of citrus fruit. But getting enough calcium is tough, especially in the case of the age groups from eleven to twenty-four years whose calcium RDA the federal government has recently increased from 800 to 1,200 milligrams. One eight-ounce glass of milk, whether it is whole milk, low-fat, or nonfat, contains approximately 200 milligrams of calcium, or 16 percent of this group's need. Often, high-calcium foods are high in fat, and some people are unable to eat calcium foods due to lactose intolerance. The trend to fortify foods with calcium, such as orange juice, can help. Choose foods wisely, as often as possible, to meet requirements.

Centrum is a good all-around vitamin supplement that is available at local pharmacies as well as in many supermarkets. Some generic supermarket brands that are one-a-day vitamin-mineral supplements are also fine. Beware of "stress" formulas, even if you live a stressful

---

* RDA: Recommended Daily Dietary Allowances are created by the Food and Nutrition Board, National Academy of Sciences, National Research Council. They are designed for the maintenance of good nutrition.

life. While the acute stress of surgical procedures or injuries can increase calorie and nutrient needs, psychological stresses such as fear, anger, and tension generally fall into the category of normal stresses of daily living and do not substantially increase nutrient needs. There is some evidence to support the need to increase potassium during stress, but this is best done by eating more fruits and vegetables—two of the best, easiest "fast foods."

Avoid supplements with megadoses of vitamins and minerals that are greater than 100 percent of the U.S. RDA. Vitamin A, for example, has become popular because of its role in helping prevent cancer and to improve acne conditions. As a consequence, its popularity has made over-the-counter vitamin A supplements readily available. In large amounts, however, this vitamin functions as a drug, and should be taken only under the supervision of a physician.

The rating scale will help you select fast foods that will improve your diet's vitamin/mineral balance.

HOW TO USE THE FAST-FOOD RATING SCALE

The purpose of the rating sale is to provide an answer to those food and eating questions in a simple, easy-to-understand way. It explains why fast-food burgers and fries, for example, cannot be totally dismissed as "junk" food. You *can* get nutrients (zinc, iron, protein, et cetera) from them as well as from the so-called natural foods. In fact, a candy bar and a burger may have more nutrients than an apple or an orange. *But* the score is lower for the burger and candy because they have more fat, calories, and no fiber. For instance, McDonald's Big Mac rates a 3, losing points because of fat, saturated fat, sodium, and low fiber, whereas the orange rates a 10. The idea is to look for the choice with the highest rating when you go to a fast-food restaurant, or make selections in a deli or from the frozen foods. And remember, *quantity* can make any choice right or wrong. Eating a *lot* of moderately fat food is worse than eating just a little very high fat food.

There is no perfect score. Yogurt, for example, gets a 9, losing 1 point for fiber. Of course we don't expect to have fiber in yogurt. That is why we must eat a mixture of foods. The real goal, obviously, is to eat more top-rated foods, the 8s, 9s, and 10s, and eat less of the lower-rated foods, especially the 1s through 5s. There are no "good" and "bad" foods, there are only "good" and "bad" diets. Even high-fat foods can be a part of a healthy diet *if* they are balanced with low-fat food choices.

There is also no specific score that you must achieve. The rating scale empowers you to make better choices, quickly and without difficult calculations. Making the choices is up to you. Each time that you select a food with a higher number than the foods you normally consume, you'll be making progress and improving your health *without* having to spend any extra time at it.

I suggest that you keep a chart for two weeks, longer if you like, to allow you to evaluate your choices and your progress. Before deciding to eat a particular food, check its rating; if it's low, ask yourself how many other low-rated foods you've eaten at this meal, during this day, and during this week. Do you have any problems with cholesterol or excess weight that would make a particular nutrient your special concern? Check the components of the rating of the foods you're considering. Ask yourself where you can make improvements. Plan ahead. Set your own goals. If *all* your meal choices are low-rated, tackle one meal at a time. Get its rating up by making some different choices before moving on to make improvements in the next meal. On those days when you slide into the "depths" (say 3 or 4) at breakfast and lunch, you can help pull yourself back up by getting a 9 or 10 at dinner.

For those who absolutely require structured goals, I suggest aiming, gradually, for the following:

- Make 65 percent of your food selections 8 or higher (18 out of 28 meals or snacks in a week).
- Allow 25 percent of your selections to fall into the 5 to 7 range (7 out of 28 meals or snacks in a week).
- Hold to 10 percent those selections with scores between 1 and 4 (3 out of 28 meals or snacks in a week).

AN IMPORTANT NOTE ABOUT THE RATING SCALE

I have listed the number of grams of fat and saturated fat for each food, but the healthfulness of fat grams and saturated fat grams is primarily dependent on their relationship to total calories. The percentage of calories from fat rather than the actual number of fat grams determines when the fat gram listing is a reason for losing points and is therefore in boldface. For example: Chicken chow mein contains 15 grams of fat and 380 calories, and loses points because the percentage of calories from fat is almost 40 percent. Pizza has 17 grams of fat for 685 calories and does not lose points for its fat content because it has a lower *percentage* of fat, just under 25 percent. Although your goal should be to keep your percentage of calories derived from fat to less than 30, that does not mean that every food must derive less than 30 percent of its calories from fat. It is your total daily grams of fat, rather than the amount of fat in a single food, that is the key to keeping fat intake at the recommended level. (See the chart on suggested fat intake per day on page 17.)

THE TYPICAL FAST-FOOD DIET VERSUS THE NEW FAST-FOOD DIET

One of my clients, Jim, is a twenty-four-year-old owner of a catering business truck. He drives a route each day, stopping at various work sites and office buildings. Hungry (or bored) workers run out to the truck to buy food and snacks. His truck actually includes a deli and grill, and Jim has a cook on board to prepare the food.

Jim was overweight and complained of low energy. When I looked at his daily diet, I saw he was skipping breakfast, eating a burger and fries for lunch, drinking soft drinks all day long, and consuming candy bars as snacks. At night, Jim and his housemates all went their own way for dinner. Jim would generally order a pepperoni pizza and eat at least half of it one night and half the next night. Jim's was the typical fast-food eating style.

Jim dropped seven pounds in the first week by doing some very simple things:

• He switched from the burger to tuna or turkey sandwiches for lunch.
• The truck began using light mayonnaise (none of the customers noticed the difference).
• He ordered—and ate—a salad along with the pizza in the evening, which immediately reduced his pizza intake.
• He replaced cola with mineral water.

I also came up with a list of seven alternative lunches and dinners for Jim.

I was able to take Jim's overall diet from a 2 or 3 to a 5 or a 6. The improvement in Jim's energy level has been enormous. Now, instead of sitting in front of the TV eating, Jim takes a long walk. He is even learning to scuba dive. And his customers are getting healthier fast-food fare, too!

So, let's move on. It's time for breakfast. You can begin putting the rating scale to work in your own life . . . starting now!

CHAPTER · 3

THE FAST-FOOD BREAKFAST

SKIPPING BREAKFAST CAN BE FATTENING (AND OTHERWISE HAZARDOUS TO YOUR HEALTH)

Many people who live fast skip breakfast. Their reasons may be that they lack the time, or that they don't like breakfast foods. Perhaps they simply can't face food in the morning because they ate too much the night before. Besides, they rationalize, skipping breakfast saves calories. Give them a cup of coffee, and they are back on the daily treadmill. Perhaps they will grab a doughnut or a muffin at a mid-morning meeting or break. Chances are, they won't think about food until their stomachs start growling around lunchtime, reminding them to eat.

But skipping breakfast is a big mistake, so finds endocrinologist C. Wayne Callaway of George Washington University in Washington, D.C. His research reveals that those who skip breakfast are likely to have *more* body fat, gain more weight (or lose less), and have high blood cholesterol levels. Irregular eating can lead to wide fluctuations in blood sugar and insulin levels, which can affect energy during the day. Breakfast skippers typically consume more fat and dietary cholesterol, fewer essential vitamins and minerals, and less dietary fiber.

Mom was right when she told the kids that breakfast was the most important meal of the day. New information to support this old claim may even convince Mom to eat breakfast herself.

First, eating breakfast helps to *distribute calories evenly* throughout the day. Breakfast skippers generally eat more of their calories late in the day, often as a single meal at dinnertime. That's not in their best interest. And there is scientific evidence to prove it. Dr. Callaway's research indicates that if you eat just one big meal a day, you will burn fewer calories than someone who eats the same amount of food spread out over breakfast, lunch, dinner, and snacks. Each meal we eat sparks a little increase in the rate at which we burn calories. This is called the "thermic effect" of food. The habit of "nibbling" throughout the day, rather than "gorging" at one large meal, has also been shown to lower insulin and cholesterol levels.*

Skipping breakfast also makes losing weight hard. One study measured weight loss when people were given all their daily calories in the morning rather than at night. Despite eating the same amount of food, the morning eaters lost more weight than the evening eaters. It appears that food eaten earlier in the day is more likely to be used for energy than to be stored as fat.

Breakfast also helps people control weight by regulating hunger. Many overweight individuals who come to me for counseling report that they skip breakfast, eat little or no lunch, then are out of control at dinner, followed by frequent snacking right up until bedtime. If they eat breakfast, they initially report that this makes them hungrier all day long. But, in fact, this hunger is not a response to breakfast but rather the deprivation of the day before. Once they consistently space their meals throughout the day, never allowing their hunger to veer out of control, they stop overeating at night, wake up hungry for breakfast and are *less* hungry later in the day.

Breakfast is good preventive medicine from the psychological point of view, as well. Have a bite to eat in the morning to avoid the feeling of starvation at lunchtime. Extreme hunger helps many justify making poor lunch choices—a giant burger and fries, for example. On the other hand, if you had eaten a bagel midmorning, you could be satisfied with soup and salad at lunchtime. The same rationale follows at dinner time. Having eaten half or even two-thirds of your day's calorie requirement by 5:00 P.M., you are, in a way, "protected" from hunger, and will be satisfied with the remainder of your calorie requirement at dinner—for example a salad and one or two slices of pizza rather than diving right into the pizza and eating 4 or 5 slices—a possible 500-calorie difference.

We can't ignore that stress is also a factor when it comes to overeating after a long, hard day at work. But don't forget that exercise is a much more effective way to reduce stress than eating—with some terrific benefits. If you have eaten wisely during the day, beginning with breakfast, you are far more likely to have the energy to go out for

* David Jenkins, et al., "Nibbling vs. Gorging: Metabolic Advantages of Increased Meal Frequency, *New England Journal of Medicine* 321, no. 14 (1989): 929–34.

a walk before dinner. As you can see, breakfast is a *key* meal. Its beneficial effects are felt all day long.

A GOOD FAST-FOOD BREAKFAST

The basic fast-food breakfast should include a protein, a complex carbohydrate, and a fruit. *Balance* is most important—too little protein may make you hungry, too much carbohydrate can make you sleepy. Most of all, too much food will slow you down. One client came to me, a very bright thirty-one-year-old medical technologist, complaining that she was so careful about all the foods she ate—choosing whole grains, low-fat dairy products, and the leanest of meats, supplemented by fruits and vegetables. She was obsessed with what she ate, but as a consequence, ate too much and remained twenty pounds overweight and was very tired throughout the day, too tired to exercise, she said.

I'm not saying you need to get a calculator out to count calories, but *control* the amount of food that you eat. Consider your activity level. If you walk or jog or swim before breakfast, or if your work is physical, take that into consideration. If you are going to an office and will be sitting in a chair all day, you need to eat less. Eat the right amount of calories to fuel your energy needs until lunch and you will have more energy and be more likely to maintain or achieve your proper weight. Now let's look at the individual breakfast components.

Complex Carbohydrates

Build your breakfast around a good source of complex carbohydrate—a not-too-processed starch, such as an unprocessed form of wheat, corn, oat, rye, rice, or other grain. Typical breakfast foods that contain these are cereals and whole-grain breads. Their value is in their chemical structure, which ensures a more gradual breakdown to glucose—the ultimate fuel, provided in a steady state without the bouncing blood sugar syndrome of doughnuts and soft drinks. And what a great source of fiber, which not only contributes to the sensation of fullness but also assures the normal functioning of the bowels.

Limit fat on bread or muffins to one teaspoon of butter or margarine *or* one tablespoon of cream cheese (low-fat if possible), *or* one tablespoon of jam or jelly (a great *substitute* for butter or margarine). Limit yourself to one to three servings of bread. If you are a large man, you can eat more; if you are a small woman, you should eat less. One serving is one slice of bread, half a bagel or English muffin, one cup of uncooked cereal, or a half cup of cooked cereal.

Protein

Just the word *protein* commands respect. It's true that every cell is made at least in part of protein, and that protein is an essential nutrient. Protein also helps to keep you alert (without the side effects of caffeine), and it will stave off hunger. Approximately one-third of your daily protein intake should be at breakfast. This amounts to 15 to 20 grams, which is easily met by eating the simple cereal-milk-toast-fruit breakfast.

Be aware, however, that when it comes to protein, more is not always better. *Too much* protein is often accompanied by too much fat, cholesterol, and calories, and not enough fiber, as in the ham (or bacon) and egg breakfast. Clearly a regular bacon and eggs breakfast must be considered "history"—people who live fast must make their calories work for them and not against them.

Fruit or Juice

Fruit is a great source of fiber, vitamins, and minerals. It is easy to fit fruit into breakfast. Put a few strawberries on your cereal or a sliced banana on your peanut butter toast. A slice of melon is a treat. If your stomach can't handle acidic fruit first thing in the morning, take an orange with you when you leave the house and eat the fruit later in the day.

Although it's true that fruit is a significant part of a healthy breakfast, ignore those claims that you should eat nothing *but* fruit until noon. Promoters of this rationale say "eating food in the wrong combinations will make it impossible for your body to digest your food, leading to weight gain." However, they never explain how undigested food that doesn't get to your bloodstream and isn't converted to energy or fat can increase weight.

Of course, there is nothing *wrong* with eating only fruit in the morning if, for example, you ate a heavy meal late the night before and don't feel like eating your usual breakfast. But eating only fruit for breakfast won't help you lose weight unless you decrease your total daily calories. (Obviously, an orange or a banana will provide fewer calories than a doughnut or a sweet roll.)

Coffee or Tea?

If you get that feeling of satisfaction from a hot drink in the morning, you'll be glad to know that the ill-health effects of caffeine seem to be disproved by one study as soon as they are proven by another. Still, I don't recommend a lot of caffeine. Limit caffeine consumption to the amount in one or two cups of coffee or tea a day, and add low-fat milk instead of cream if you add anything. Consider having other beverages with your breakfast, such as skim milk, buttermilk, water, or fruit juice.

THE FAST-FOOD DIET CAN BRING BREAKFAST BACK INTO YOUR LIFE

Start at the Store

Smart shopping, along with careful planning, is the key to getting breakfast back into your life. Review the rating chart of breakfasts at the end of this chapter, try to select those with the higher ratings (see preceding chapter for guidelines), and make your list. Select a variety of cereals—flakes, biscuits, bran. Choose a few different breads to prevent boredom, such as bagels, English muffins, pita, rye, or wheat bread. These can be frozen if necessary, then popped into the toaster or microwave oven for a quick, hot breakfast. Frozen whole-grain waffles are also a good quick choice: just toast them, add jelly instead of butter, and you have a hot breakfast.

If you shop once a week, perishable items should stay fresh and wholesome until your next trip. Perhaps you will need to pick up a carton of milk, fresh fish, or a few bananas during the week, easy to do at a small market on your trip home, rather than making a special trip to the supermarket midweek.

If You Don't Have Time

If time is the major obstacle between you and breakfast, be sure to choose a breakfast that requires little or no preparation. Mornings tend to be hectic, sleeping past the alarm, then maybe hopping on the exercise bike or going for a jog, getting kids ready for school, followed by a quick shower, and getting dressed for work. The breakfasts described in this chapter should provide some quick solutions for those with hectic schedules.

Take It with You

There is no need to eat immediately on arising. In fact, we can redefine breakfast as "something to eat before lunch" rather than "something to eat before work." If you leave for work at six or seven in the morning, or if you simply can't face food in the morning, you may want to have your breakfast *after* you arrive at your destination. As long as you eat midmorning and don't hold off until lunchtime, all of the benefits of breakfast will still be yours.

Even if you do eat at home, you may need a midmorning snack to avoid becoming overly hungry at lunchtime, which leads to overeating lunch, and as a consequence, being tired in the midafternoon. Why not carry food with you to eat later? A plain bagel and a banana fit nicely into a plastic bag. When midmorning choices are vending machine candy bars or cafeteria doughnuts, you will be glad you have foods that taste good and give you energy rather than take it away.

Stop and Buy Breakfast

If you are in a real hurry, stop at a bagel shop or deli along the way and pick up a toasted bagel with a small amount of cream cheese or jelly and juice. A plain fresh bagel will be easy to eat en route, and a deli will be as fast or faster than standing in line at a fast-food restaurant. Convenience markets, such as AM-PM mini-mart or the 7-Eleven–type stores, may offer yogurt, crackers stuffed with peanut butter or cheese, bran muffins, juice, low-fat milk, and often fresh fruit.

If you decide to eat breakfast at a fast-food restaurant, the choice may be a compromise in good nutrition. Granted, you can hold the egg sandwich in one hand while you drive with the other, but if you truly have a busy day ahead, this is not a good way to start out. And in any case, ask yourself: is this really faster than a bowl of cereal or toast at home? (If you do pick up your breakfast at fast-food outlets, check our ratings of their breakfast offerings at the end of this chapter, with more detailed analysis in chapter 8.)

Keep a Stash at the Office

For those days when you don't have breakfast before work, keep a few items at the office. No refrigeration is needed for fruit, peanut butter*, raisins, and crackers. If you do have a refrigerator, take advantage of it, and keep an inventory on hand of fruit-flavored, low-fat yogurt, cheese or cottage cheese, V-8 juice, and fresh fruits. The only problem is that your fellow employees may find your healthy foods more appealing than their own higher-calorie alternatives. The healthy-eating trend finds many people aware and interested in eating wisely but without appealing foods at hand that will help them break away from their old habits. One person in an office can stimulate new ideas, without becoming a crusader, and create a much healthier set of alternatives for everyone who uses the office refrigerator.

Allow two weeks to retrain yourself to the habit of breakfast. In-

---

*Although peanut butter by the jarful provides too much total fat and calories, a tablespoon or two on crackers, whole-grain bread, or a banana offers a good source of monounsaturated fat with no cholesterol; the old-fashioned unhydrogenated brands offer the least saturated fats, which tend to raise cholesterol in the blood.

creased energy and enhanced weight control will be your motivation. After a few months, you may find that you wouldn't dream of starving yourself until noon—and then gorging later.

Potential problem: What happens if you do eat breakfast and then are confronted with an unexpected "meal" at a meeting? Or perhaps someone brings in something special from home to share at a coffee break. Forget the rationale that if you don't eat it you will offend someone. That's their problem; don't let it become yours. If you eat breakfast and this unexpected snack, as well, that's two breakfasts, and that's probably too much unless you ran a marathon before work. Don't let people and pressure make you fail at your efforts to eat smart and feel better. It's not worth it, and it's not necessary. Simply say, "No, thank you, I already ate breakfast." No explanation is necessary.

NUTRITIONAL ANALYSES OF SOME SIMPLE, FAST BREAKFASTS

Many people eat the same thing for breakfast most of the time, particularly during the week, with a variation on the weekend—either something special at home that requires a bit more preparation, or perhaps a brunch in a restaurant. Here are nutritional analyses of several common breakfasts, including some of the best and some of the worst choices, to help you compare the different options.

No-Preparation Breakfasts

There are endless choices and combinations of "instant" breakfasts. The best approach is to enjoy a variety of grains and be sparing with what you put on the bread and cereal. Try eating your bagel or toast dry or with minimal fat. Our guidelines suggest one teaspoon of margarine or one tablespoon of light cream cheese, peanut butter, or jelly or jam. A good rule of thumb is to put it on and then *scrape it off*, leaving a thin layer for flavor. Using *nonfat* or *low-fat* milk on cereal rather than whole milk or cream also saves fat calories, with the same amount of calcium and protein.

QUICK BREAKFASTS

QUICK BREAKFASTS	Rating	Calories	Fat (g)	Saturated Fat (g)	Cholesterol (mg)	Sodium (mg)	Fiber (g)
1 oz. recommended cereal (shredded wheat), ½ c. low-fat milk, 1 banana, & 1 slice wheat toast	10	329	4	3	12	220	8.5
1 c. orange juice, 1 slice wheat toast, 1 tbsp. peanut butter, & 1 banana	10	302	10	2	2	240	6.4
1 oz. recommended cereal, ½ c. low-fat milk, 1 slice wheat toast, 2 tsp. margarine, & 1 banana	10	396	12	0.5	9	309	8.5
Water bagel, 1 tbsp. cream cheese, 1 c. orange juice, & ½ c. sliced strawberries	10	345	8	3	16	244	1.5
1 c. plain nonfat yogurt, 1 slice wheat toast, 1 tbsp. peanut butter, 1 banana, & 1 c. coffee	10	383	10	2	4	392	4.5
Homemade bran muffin & 1 c. orange juice	10	230	5	1	21	176	2.5
Dunkin' Donuts bran muffin & 1 c. orange juice*	9	460	13	4.7	12	593	>1.5
Plain cake doughnut & 1 c. coffee†	5	112	**6**	1	10	147	**0.1**
Fancy Danish & 1 c. coffee*†	1	364	**18**	—	—	340	**<1.5**

* LOSES ADDITIONAL POINT DUE TO HIGH SUGAR CONTENT.

† LOSES ADDITIONAL POINTS DUE TO LOW VITAMIN AND MINERAL CONTENT.

NOTE: BOLDFACE NUMBERS INDICATE NUTRITIONAL FACTOR THAT DETRACTS FROM FOOD'S NUTRITIONAL VALUE (see the note on page 22).

This chart gives you several options. You may be surprised to know that you can maintain a diet that is 30 percent fat—a considerable improvement over the standard American diet—while using low-fat milk and margarine on bread. The score still comes out to be a 10. On the other hand, if you choose to limit your fat intake to a very rigorous 10 percent, then you must stay with non-fat milk and dry toast. This may be appropriate for someone who is attempting weight loss (although it is not the *only* diet that will support weight loss), or someone who is trying to reverse the buildup of atherosclerotic plaque—or in laymen's terms "trying to unclog arteries."

Weekend Breakfasts

Weekends present a change of routine for many of us. If there is time, make your own pancakes, waffles, or French toast using one of my nutritious recipes (see Chapter 10). They are made with less fat and more fiber and can be served with a high-fiber fruit and low-fat yogurt, or a reduced-calorie syrup or jelly, or less of the real maple syrup. You might have guessed by now that bacon and eggs are near the bottom of the list on the rating scale. Complex carbohydrates are the way to go if you want to maintain an active, healthy lifestyle that will let you look and feel your best.

WEEKEND BREAKFASTS	Rating	Calories	Fat (g)	Saturated Fat (g)	Cholesterol (mg)	Sodium (mg)	Fiber (g)
1 c. cooked oatmeal, ¼ c. low-fat milk, 1 tsp. brown sugar, 1 slice wheat toast, 1 tsp. margarine, & 1 c. orange juice	10	453	9	2	5	242	5.3
1 slice homemade French toast, 1 tbsp. syrup, ½ c. orange juice, & ½ c. low-fat milk*	8	331	9	1	9	357	0
1 plain homemade pancake, ½ c. low-fat milk, & 1 tbsp. syrup*†	7	183	4	2	29	259	0
2 fried eggs, 1 slice wheat toast, 2 pats butter, 1 tbsp. jam, ½ c. orange juice, 2 slices bacon, & 1 c. hash brown potatoes*	3	806	**50**	**21**	**525**	**766**	1.5
2 plain homemade pancakes, ½ c. orange juice, 1 tbsp. butter, 2 tbsp. syrup, & 2 sausage patties*	2	543	**32**	**16**	**120**	**1182**	0
2 fried eggs, 2 biscuits, ½ c. grits, 2 oz. ham, ½ c. gravy & 1 c. tea†	2	588	**30.5**	**10.4**	**484**	**1854**	0.3

* LOSES ADDITIONAL POINT DUE TO HIGH SUGAR CONTENT.
† LOSES ADDITIONAL POINTS DUE TO LOW VITAMIN AND MINERAL CONTENT.
NOTE: BOLDFACE NUMBERS INDICATE NUTRITIONAL FACTOR THAT DETRACTS FROM FOOD'S NUTRITIONAL VALUE (see the note on page 22).

New breakfast entrées offered by fast-food restaurants are at last expanding our choices. McDonald's has added a nonfat apple bran muffin to its breakfast line-up. One muffin contains 190 calories and no fat. McDonald's has also switched to one-percent low-fat milk, which is better than the two-percent low-fat milk. Good for you, McDonald's!

Burger King's new alternative to its 500 calorie cheese danish (with 36 grams of fat) is the mini-muffin. The raisin—oat bran flavor tastes pretty good. If you choose these muffins, be aware that they are small, and six are considered one serving size, providing 320–380 calories and 13–22 grams of fat.

Commercial Fast-Food Breakfasts

Think of yourself as side-tracking from your new breakfast routine if you choose to eat the fast-food restaurant egg-ham sandwiches. As much as we try to bend the rules and rearrange choices, we must be aware that these are poor choices because of their high fat and cholesterol content. Still, the typical breakfast sandwiches are reviewed in the chart below so you can see how they compare with one another and with other choices. For a complete list of the breakfast offerings at specific fast-food restaurants, and the ratings, see Chapter 8.

FAST-FOOD BREAKFASTS	Rating	Calories	Fat (g)	Saturated Fat (g)	Cholesterol (mg)	Sodium (mg)	Fiber (g)
McDonald's Apple Bran Muffin & 6 oz. orange juice*	9	270	0	0	0	230	>1.5
Toasted English muffin, 2 tsp. margarine, 1 tbsp. jam, & 6 oz. orange juice*	8	362	9	2	0	506	<1
Hardee's 3 Pancakes w/syrup and margarine/butter blend*	7	485	6	1	20	**935**	<1.5
McDonald's Egg McMuffin, & 6 oz. orange juice	7	370	11.2	3.8	**226**	**740**	<1
Jack in the Box's Breakfast Jack & 6 oz. orange juice	6	412	**14**	0.1	**182**	**1039**	<1
1 scrambled egg with 1 oz. ham in 1 pita bread & 6 oz. orange juice	5	354	**13**	**5**	**262**	**760**	0.3
Croissant with 1 oz. ham, 1 oz. cheese, 1 slice bacon, 1 fried egg, & 6 oz. orange juice	3	598	**37**	**11**	**292**	**1326**	<1
1 biscuit with 1 sausage patty, 1 fried egg, 1 oz. cheese, & 6 oz. orange juice	3	481	**29**	**12**	**295**	**1081**	<1

* LOSES ADDITIONAL POINT DUE TO HIGH SUGAR CONTENT.
NOTE: BOLDFACE NUMBERS INDICATE NUTRITIONAL FACTOR THAT DETRACTS FROM FOOD'S NUTRITIONAL VALUE (see the note on page 22).

Dinner for Breakfast

If you lean toward avoiding breakfast because traditional breakfast foods are unappealing to you, then try what one of my clients does. She works the night shift as a nurse and plays two hours of tennis six days a week. In the morning, she picks up chicken chow mein from her favorite oriental restaurant and has that for breakfast. Although this is typically considered "dinner," it is a perfect combination of foods, one that gives her the protein and complex carbohydrates she needs to start her day. The chart below reviews a few "dinner" breakfasts, several of which rate 7 or higher.

DINNER FOR BREAKFAST

	Rating	Calories	Fat (g)	Saturated Fat (g)	Cholesterol (mg)	Sodium (mg)	Fiber (g)
2 oz. turkey breast on 2 slices wheat toast with romaine lettuce, tomato slice, 1 tsp. mustard, 1 apple, & 1 c. low-fat milk	10	423	5	2.6	65	288	>1.5
1 c. low-fat cottage cheese with banana, 10 peanuts, & 1 c. orange juice	9	478	12	3	10	**928**	4
2 slices cheese pizza & 1 c. orange juice	8	684	17	6.8	**113**	**1402**	3.8
1 c. chicken chow mein & 1 c. low-fat milk	6	380	**15**	**5**	**116**	**845**	>1.5
Flour tortilla or 1 slice french bread with 2 oz. cheddar cheese & 1 c. orange juice	5	427	**21**	**12**	60	358	**0**

NOTE: BOLDFACE NUMBERS INDICATE NUTRITIONAL FACTOR THAT DETRACTS FROM FOOD'S NUTRITIONAL VALUE (see the note on page 22).

TIPS ON SELECTING CEREALS

Cereal wins the prize as the number-one breakfast choice—when the right type is selected—not only because of its contribution to good nutrition, but because it is *fast*: just "pour and eat" at home, at the office, at your desk. Top your cereal with nonfat or low-fat milk and fresh fruit. Bananas are available all year round. Take advantage of fresh peaches or strawberries when they are in season. If you don't have fresh fruit, put two spoonfuls of raisins on your cereal.

You must be cautious with certain kinds of cereals. My client, Jim, loved to eat the Quaker 100% natural cereal, until he realized that his one-cup serving contained *over 4 teaspoons of fat, 7 teaspoons of sugar, and 520 calories!* Now he mixes a quarter cup of his granola with a half cup of shredded wheat and a quarter cup of Grape-Nuts. This greatly improves his choice without completely sacrificing the granola taste.

Cereal is the best alternative to bacon and eggs and it certainly beats coffee and doughnuts. It provides a great source of nutrients and fiber, and it stays with you. Since the basis of cereals is grains, and grains are naturally low in fat, most cereals are consequently low-fat foods, unless nuts, seeds, oils, or other ingredients high in fat are added.

New cereals are introduced all the time. Many contain claims such as "all natural, fortified with 100 percent of essential vitamins and minerals, no preservatives, no added sugar, and high fiber." Although these claims may be true, you must be aware of fat, calories, salt, and natural sources of sugar. To simplify your search for the best cereal, use the following guide as you check the nutrition label. You want a cereal that will deliver, *per serving*, something close to this:

☞ 4 grams of protein
2 grams of fat, *or less*
2 grams of fiber, *minimum*
200 milligrams of sodium, *or less*
3 to 4 grams of sugar or less (about 1 teaspoon of sugar in any form)

Remember, the shorter the ingredient list on your cereal box, the more nutritious the cereal is likely to be. Shredded wheat, for example, contains only "100 percent wheat." Ingredients listed first are the main ingredients; those farther down the list are present in smaller amounts.

Check the calories listed per serving size. These can range from 140 calories for a quarter cup of sugary, fatty granola or Mueslix to 60 calories for a half cup of Fiber One. The lowest-calorie cereal for the volume is unsweetened puffed wheat or rice, with two cups providing less than 100 calories. Choose a cereal you enjoy so that you will stay with it. Try to look for some kind of whole grain as the *first* ingredient listed, whether it is whole wheat, rye, corn, or oats.

Don't be fooled by claims of vitamin and mineral supplementation beyond 10 to 25 percent; they are most likely cover-ups for an overly processed grain. There is no need for 100 percent of vitamins and minerals unless cereal is the only thing you intend to eat all day. The cereal Total, for example, makes this claim, but the vitamins added to this product do not make up for nutrients and fiber lost during the process of refining the grain. Always begin with a *whole* grain.

Here are a few that I recommend:

READY-TO-EAT CEREALS WITH NO MILK

	Protein (g)	Added Sugar (g)	Fat (g)	Sodium (mg)	Fiber (g)
HIGHLY RECOMMENDED—THE BEST					
Kellogg's Bran Buds, ⅓ c.	3	**7**	1	170	8
Kellogg's Heartwise, ⅔ c.	3	**5**	1	140	5
Quaker Shredded Wheat, ⅔ c.	3	0	1	0	3
Quaker Shredded Wheat 'n Bran, ⅔ c.	3	0	1	0	4
Kellogg's Just Right w/Fiber Nuggets, ⅔ c.	2	**5**	1	200	2
Kellogg's Just Right w/Fruit & Nuts, ¾ c.	3	**9**	1	190	2
Kellogg's Mueslix Crispy Blend, ⅔ c.	4	**8**	2	140	4
Kellogg's Mueslix Golden Crunch, ½ c.	4	<4	1	55	4
Kellogg's Nutri-Grain Wheat, ⅔ c.	3	2	0	170	3
Ralston Purina Crispy Oatmeal & Raisin Chex, ¾ c.	3	<4	0.5	168	**1.7**
Ralston Purina Wheat & Raisin Chex, ¾ c.	3	<4	0.3	198	3.4

READY-TO-EAT CEREALS WITH NO MILK (continued)

	Protein (g)	Added Sugar (g)	Fat (g)	Sodium (mg)	Fiber (g)
Ralston Purina Wheat Chex, ⅔ c.	3	<4	0.7	200	3.4
100% Bran, ⅓ c.	4	<4	1.4	196	3.4
Post Raisin Bran, ½ c.	3	<4	0.4	178	3.7
Post Fruit & Fiber (avg. of flavors), ½ c.	3	<4	1	181	4.2
VERY RECOMMENDED—PRETTY GOOD					
Kellogg's All-Bran, ⅓ c.	4	**5**	1	**260**	10
Kellogg's Frosted Mini-Wheats, 1 oz. (about 4 biscuits)	3	**6**	0	0	3
General Mills Fiber One, ½ c.	**2**	0	1	140	13
Kellogg's Apple Cinnamon Squares, ½ c.	**2**	**6**	0	5	2
Kellogg's Blueberry Squares, ½ c.	**2**	**5**	0	5	3
Kellogg's Bran Flakes, ⅔ c.	3	**5**	0	**220**	5
Kellogg's Common Sense Oat Bran, ½ c.	4	**5**	1	**270**	3
Kellogg's Common Sense Oat Bran w/raisins, ½ c.	4	**5**	0	**250**	3
Kellogg's Raisin Bran, ¾ c.	3	**13**	1	**230**	5
Kellogg's Raisin Squares, ½ c.	**2**	**6**	0	0	2
Kellogg's Strawberry Squares, ½ c.	**2**	**5**	0	5	3
Post Bran Flakes, ⅔ c.	3	<4	0.4	**227**	5.6
Ralston Purina Bran Chex, ⅔ c.	3	<4	0.7	**299**	6.1
Ralston Purina Bran Flakes, ¾ c.	3	<4	0.4	**264**	3.5
General Mills Cheerios, 1¼ c.	4	<4	1.8	**290**	2
Post Grape-Nuts, ¼ c.	3	<4	0.1	188	**1.8**
General Mills Raisin Nut Bran, ½ c.	3	<4	**3**	140	3
General Mills Wheaties, 1 c.	3	<4	0.5	**270**	2
General Mills Total, 1 c.	3	<4	0.6	**280**	2
Kellogg's Fruitful Bran, ⅔ c.	3	**11**	0	**230**	5
Nutri-Grain Almond Raisin, ⅔ c.	3	**7**	2	**220**	3
RECOMMENDED—ACCEPTABLE					
Kellogg's Corn Flakes, 1 c.	**2**	2	0	**290**	**1**
Quaker Puffed Wheat Cereal, 1 c.	**2**	0	<4	0	**0.5**
Quaker Corn Bran, ⅔ c.	**2**	<4	1	**300**	5.4
Kellogg's Cracklin' Oat Bran, ½ c.	3	**7**	**4**	150	4
Ralston Purina Almond Delight, ¾ c.	**2**	<4	1.6	199	**1.5**
Team Flakes, 1 c.	**2**	<4	0.5	175	**0.3**
Post Fortified Oat Flakes, ⅔ c.	6	<4	0.5	**247**	**0.8**
General Mills Crispy Wheats & Raisins, ¾ c.	**2**	<4	0.5	180	**1.3**
Ralston Purina Corn Chex, 1 c.	**2**	<4	0.2	**293**	**1.1**
Ralston Purina Rice Chex, 1⅛ c.	**2**	<4	0.3	**252**	**0.5**
General Mills Honey Nut Cheerios, ¾ c.	3	**>4**	0.7	**250**	2
General Mills Kix, 1½ c.	3	**>4**	0.7	**290**	**0.4**
Post Grape-Nut Flakes, ⅞ c.	3	<4	0.8	158	**1.9**

READY-TO-EAT CEREALS WITH NO MILK (continued)

	Protein (g)	Added Sugar (g)	Fat (g)	Sodium (mg)	Fiber (g)
LIFE (regular and cinnamon), ⅔ c.	5	>4	2	180	**0.9**
Raisin LIFE, ⅔ c.	5	>4	2	200	**0.9**
Kellogg's Nut & Honey Crunch, ⅔ c.	**2**	9	1	200	—
Kellogg's Product 19, 1 c.	3	3	0	**320**	1
Kellogg's Rice Krispies, 1 c.	**2**	3	0	**290**	—
Kellogg's Special K, 1 c.	6	3	0	**230**	—

NOTE: BOLDFACE NUMBERS INDICATE NUTRITONAL FACTOR THAT DETRACTS FROM FOOD'S NUTRITIONAL VALUE (see the note on page 22).

There are some popular favorites I can't recommend because they are too high in sugar (around 50 percent of weight). They include Sugar Smacks, Apple Jacks, Froot Loops, Cocoa Pebbles, Frosted Flakes, Cap'n Crunch, Lucky Charms, Honeycomb, and Cookie Crisp. All granola-type cereals are too high in fat as well as sugar to be recommended.

ALL BREAKFASTS

	Rating	Calories	Fat (g)	Saturated Fat (g)	Cholesterol (mg)	Sodium (mg)	Fiber (g)
1 oz. recommended cereal (shredded wheat), ½ c. low-fat milk, 1 banana, & 1 slice wheat toast	10	329	4	3	12	220	8.5
1 oz. recommended cereal, ½ c. low-fat milk, 1 banana, wheat toast, & 2 tsp. margarine	10	396	12	0.5	9	309	8.5
Water bagel, 1 tsp. cream cheese, 1 c. orange juice, & ½ c. sliced strawberries	10	369	7	3	16	244	1.5
1 c. orange juice, 1 slice wheat toast, 1 tbsp. peanut butter, & 1 banana	10	302	10	2	2	292	6.4
1 c. plain nonfat yogurt, 1 slice wheat toast, 1 tbsp. peanut butter, 1 banana, & 1 c. orange juice	10	389	10	2	4	388	4.5
1 c. cooked oatmeal, ¼ c. low-fat milk, 1 tsp. brown sugar, 1 slice wheat toast, 1 tsp. margarine, & 1 c. orange juice	10	453	9	2	5	242	5.3
2 oz. turkey breast on 2 slices wheat toast with romaine lettuce, tomato slice, 1 tsp. mustard, 1 apple, & 1 c. low-fat milk	10	423	5	2.6	65	288	>1.5
Homemade bran muffin & 1 c. orange juice	10	230	5	1	21	176	2.5
Dunkin' Donuts bran muffin & 1 c. orange juice*	9	460	13	4.7	12	593	>1.5
McDonald's Apple Bran Muffin & 6 oz. orange juice*	9	270	0	0	0	230	>1.5

BREAKFASTS (continued)

	Rating	Calories	Fat (g)	Saturated Fat (g)	Cholesterol (mg)	Sodium (mg)	Fiber (g)
1 c. low-fat cottage cheese w/banana, 10 peanuts, & 1 c. orange juice	9	478	12	5	10	**928**	4
1 slice homemade French toast, 1 tbsp. syrup, ½ c. orange juice, ½ c. milk*	8	331	9	1	9	357	**0**
Toasted English muffin, 2 tsp. margarine, 1 tbsp. jam, & 6 oz. orange juice*	8	362	9	2	0	506	**<1**
2 slices cheese pizza & 1 c. orange juice	8	684	17	6.8	**113**	**1402**	3.8
1 plain homemade pancake, ½ c. low-fat milk, & 1 tbsp. syrup*†	7	183	4	2	29	259	**0**
McDonald's Egg McMuffin & 6 oz. orange juice	7	370	11.2	3.8	**226**	**740**	**<1**
Hardee's Three Pancakes w/syrup & margarine/butter blend*	7	485	6	1	20	**955**	**<1.5**
1 c. homemade chicken chow mein & 1 c. low-fat milk	6	380	**15**	**5**	**116**	**845**	>1.5
Plain cake doughnut & 1 c. coffee*†	5	112	**6**	1	10	147	**0.1**
Jack in the Box's Breakfast Jack & 6 oz. orange juice	5	387	**13**	**5.2**	**203**	**871**	**<1**
Scrambled egg with 1 oz. ham in pita bread & 1 c. orange juice	5	354	**13**	**5**	**262**	**760**	**0.3**
Flour tortilla with 2 oz. Cheddar cheese & 1. c. orange juice	5	427	**21**	**12**	60	358	**0**
Croissant with 1 oz. ham, 1 oz. cheese, 1 slice bacon, 1 egg, 6 oz. orange juice	3	598	**37**	**11**	**292**	**1326**	**<1**
Biscuit with 1 sausage patty, 1 egg, 1 oz. cheese, & 6 oz. orange juice	3	481	**29**	**12**	**295**	**1081**	**<1**
2 fried eggs, 1 slice wheat toast, 2 tsp. butter, 1 tbsp. jam, ½ c. orange juice, 2 slices bacon, & 1 c. hash brown potatoes	3	806	**50**	**21**	**525**	**766**	1.5
2 plain homemade pancakes, ½ c. orange juice, 2 tbsp. syrup, 1 tbsp. butter, & 2 sausage patties	2	543	**32**	**16**	**120**	**1182**	**0**
2 fried eggs, 2 biscuits, ½ c. grits, 2 oz. ham, ½ c. gravy & 1 c. tea	2	588	**30.5**	**10.4**	**484**	**1854**	**0.3**
Fancy Danish & 1 c. coffee*†	1	364	**18**	—	—	340	**<1.5**

* LOSES ADDITIONAL POINT DUE TO HIGH SUGAR CONTENT.

† LOSES ADDITONAL POINTS DUE TO LOW VITAMIN AND MINERAL CONTENT.

NOTE: BOLDFACE NUMBERS INDICATE NUTRITIONAL FACTOR THAT DETRACTS FROM FOOD'S NUTRITIONAL VALUE (see the note on page 22).

CHAPTER · 4

THE FAST-FOOD LUNCH

THE LUNCH CHALLENGE

Lunch is often the biggest challenge for people who are trying to manage their weight and eat healthy food with limited time. This is partly due to the fact that lunch is the meal most frequently eaten away from home.

In addition to being a challenge, the lunch meal is very important to success on the job. The right lunch can make the difference between a productive afternoon and falling asleep at your desk. Those who live fast, and who must meet heavy demands in their jobs, need a lunch that works for them, not against them. Make the right lunch choices for maximum brain power by considering the following rules:

First rule: Eat sparingly. Limit your calories at lunch, and you'll be surprised how much better you feel and perform. Joe is one of my clients, an investment counselor who entertains his Mexican clients with their customary three-to-four hour lavish lunches. The meal usually includes six or seven courses, beginning with appetizers, soup, salad, richly sauced pasta, meat entrée, vegetables, bread, desserts, several bottles of wine, and finally, Cognac. Joe explained that these lunches were important to establishing rapport with his clients, so that he could gain their confidence in his ability to profitably invest their money in the United States. But as important as the long lunches were, they were getting in the way of his personal priorities of weight loss and exercise. He was simply eating too much food and drinking too much alcohol. And after that, he was too tired for his daily workout of aerobics and weights at the gym.

Joe realized that he needed to manage this problem, so that it wouldn't manage him. He accepted much of my advice and soon ate soup only when it was a minestrone, vegetable, or broth-based soup. He chose a char-grilled fish as his entrée whenever possible. He ate his lightly dressed salad, pushed aside any cheese, and ignored dessert. He began to ask the waiter to bring him half the normal portion of the entrée and filled up on vegetables. He limited his wine to one glass instead of two and sipped on mineral water instead. For all the courses, from soup to salad to entrée to dessert, he stopped short of devouring all the food in front of him; instead, he focused on his business at hand. These changes, not noticeable to his clients, cut calories by two-thirds from about 2,500 to 800. And when the meal was over and his clients were headed for their siestas, Joe was off to the gym.

Second rule: Approach lunch with hunger already in check. The best way to do this, as previously noted, is to *eat breakfast*. You may also want to have a midmorning snack: an apple, banana, or a package of raisins, for example, that can easily be stored in your desk. Have a planned midafternoon snack waiting. (See chapter 6 for more ideas on snacks.)

Third rule: Balance the amount of carbohydrates, protein, and fat in a way that works to your advantage: three to four ounces of protein; 100 or 200 calories worth of bread, rice, pasta or other starch; and a limited amount of fat. Avoid rich fatty foods such as cream soups, meat-dominant hot dishes, or too much creamy dressing on salads or too much butter or mayonnaise on bread. Choose a fruit for dessert for 100 or 200 calories, containing no fat, rather than a dessert with 200 to 500 calories, 75 percent of them derived from fat. If you have more of a sweet tooth and want a dessert, choose a *small* cookie, or share a dessert with a friend.

SOLVING THE PROBLEM OF LUNCH

Fast-Food Restaurant

Here are the options for the fast-food lunch. *All* can be used without compromising your nutritional objectives. We suggest that you shop around your neighborhood to find all the right places.

This choice seems like a natural since there are so many of them, they're fast, and, let's face it, the taste isn't all that bad. The problem is, unless you're careful, it's easy to get too many calories. The typical quarter-pound burger along with fries and milk shake will deliver

1,200 to 1,500 calories—that's enough calories for the entire day for a woman who is relatively small, and half to three-quarters of the calories needed by the average man. *That's too many.* In addition, most of the calories are coming from fat (often saturated), and fiber is negligible.

Clearly, a chicken sandwich has the potential to be a better choice, at 300–400 calories. They vary, however, and the list below reveals their fat and calorie content.

	FAT (G)	CALORIES
Jack in the Box Chicken Fajita Pita (without cheese)	8	292
McDonald's Grilled Chicken Breast Sandwich	6.5	304
Hardee's Grilled Chicken Sandwich	9	310
Wendy's Grilled Chicken Sandwich	13	340
Burger King Broiler Chicken Sandwich	18	379
McDonald's McChicken Sandwich	29	490

McDonald's new packaged carrot and celery sticks are a great addition to their menu. Don't forget Wendy's chili, a good choice that has been around for a while, providing 7 grams of fat in a 9 ounce portion. Salads and or salad bars are available at all the major fast-food restaurants. It's great to see these establishments meeting the consumer demand for healthier fast food. For a complete review of the new fast-food offerings, see pages 129–150.

Mexican fast food is another option. Order plain burritos that are not fried, and skip the cheese and toppings, such as sour cream and avocado. My favorite is the chicken burrito: a corn tortilla with chicken, lettuce, and tomato. A flour or corn tortilla meets our lunch objectives: moderate protein and carbohydrate, low fat.

Remember to eat sparingly at fast-food restaurants. Instead of the big—the Whopper, the Super, et cetera—choose the standard or the small. Supplement with a salad and low-fat milk (in place of a shake) and you'll cut your fast-food calories in half and get twice the fiber, vitamins A and C, and calcium. You'll leave with a comfortable feeling, too. Frequent the outlets that offer baked potato instead of french fries, and then top the potato with *one* tablespoon of sour cream, or a sprinkle of Parmesan cheese instead of two tablespoons plus cheese, bacon, and other fatty offerings. Instead of shakes or soft drinks, look for low-fat shakes or order low-fat milk, tea, or diet soda. Keep asking for things like broiled fish and chicken, fruit juice, and salads and when they are available, *choose them*—it's *your* demand that creates the market.

Review the fast-food charts in Chapter 8 to find the choices that best meet your needs. Here is a brief overview of a few fast foods.

FAST-FOOD LUNCHES	Rating	Calories	Fat (g)	Saturated Fat (g)	Cholesterol (mg)	Sodium (mg)	Fiber (g)
McDonald's Chunky Chicken Salad w/1 tbsp. Lite Vinaigrette Dressing	10	140	3.4	0.9	78	230	>1.5
Wendy's plain baked potato, garden salad, & 1 tbsp. low-cal Italian dressing	10	397	7	<5	0	315	>1.5
Taco Bell bean burrito w/sauce	9	357	10	2.9	9	**888**	>1.5
Domino's 2 slices cheese pizza	9	376	10	**5.5**	19	484	6.4
Wendy's chili and plain baked potato	9	490	7	2.6	45	**750**	>1.5
Carl's Jr. roast beef sandwich, side salad, & 1 tbsp. low-cal dressing	8	533	13.5	**<8**	60	**1290**	>1.5
Jack in the Box chicken fajita pita (includes lettuce, tomato, onions, & cheese)*	8	292	8	2.9	34	**704**	**<1.5**
Wendy's broccoli & cheese–stuffed potato	8	400	**16**	**2.9**	<15	455	>1.5
KFC extra-crispy drumstick†, corn on the cob, 3 oz. mashed potatoes*	7	408	**15**	4	65	584	**<1.5**
McDonald's plain hamburger & low-fat frozen yogurt cone*	6	360	10.3	**4**	40	580	**<1.5**
McDonald's plain hamburger, side salad, 1 tbsp. low-cal dressing*	6	335	**13.3**	**5.2**	78	**660**	>1.5
Burger King Whopper & regular fries	2	955	**56**	**22**	**111**	**1106**	**<1.5**

* ADD FRUIT OR FRUIT JUICE TO INCREASE RATING BY ONE POINT. LOSES ADDITIONAL POINTS DUE TO LOW VITAMIN AND MINERAL CONTENT.
† THE KEY TO THE RELATIVELY HIGH SCORE FOR THIS MEAL YOU MIGHT EXPECT TO BE HIGHER IN FAT IS THE SMALL SIZE OF THE CHICKEN: 1½ OUNCES OF MEAT ON THE DRUMSTICK.
NOTE: BOLDFACE NUMBERS INDICATE NUTRITIONAL FACTOR THAT DETRACTS FROM FOOD'S NUTRITIONAL VALUE (see the note on page 22).

Deli

Why not check your options at a deli? The sandwich is a perfect alternative to the burger. If ordered according to my guidelines, the right sandwich can provide *half* the calories of the burger with *twice* the nutritional benefits and still be just as satisfying. In an effort to compete with the speediness of the fast-food establishments, many deli counters urge their patrons to call ahead and order their sandwiches. Delis generally make sandwiches "to order" and will often oblige in special requests. Find a deli in your neighborhood, get to know them, and put their phone number in your Rolodex file or address book. When it's time for lunch, just order your usual, and the lunch problem is solved.

I urge you to use your stopwatch and actually *time* your visit to the deli. Compare it to the typical fast-food establishment and see if there is a significant difference. I'll bet it's a draw, but even if it comes out a minute or two behind, ask yourself if that difference justifies the final impact on your nutritional intake.

Here are how several "standard" deli sandwiches score:

Turkey on whole wheat with mustard, lettuce, and tomato = 10

Lean ham on whole wheat with mustard, lettuce, and tomato = 9

Roast beef on whole wheat with mustard, lettuce, and tomato = 9

Ham and cheese on whole wheat with mustard, lettuce, and tomato = 7

Vegetarian sandwich, with cheese, avocado, mayonnaise, mustard, and sprouts = 6

Sometimes deli sandwiches contain too much meat. If you know this is the case, eat only half the sandwich and save the rest. Wrap the extra meat and add to a salad, or you could use it for a sandwich the following day.

Deli lunches, other than sandwiches, require further scrutiny. Many people, unprepared to make a healthy decision and confronted by too many choices, may end up consuming more calories than they realize. However, armed with the right knowledge and persistence, those of us who want low-fat food can make good choices. Use the chart that follows to guide you.

DELI LUNCHES

	Rating	Calories	Fat (g)	Saturated Fat (g)	Cholesterol (mg)	Sodium (mg)	Fiber (g)
10 oz. rigatoni w/ham & peas & mineral water*	8	350	9	—	50	**1376**	>1.5
3½ oz. lobster or crab salad, whole wheat roll, 4 oz. low-fat fruit yogurt, & mineral water*	8	295	9	**4**	65	344	>1.5
6 oz. lasagna, ½ c. green salad w/1 tbsp. low-cal Italian dressing, & 6 oz. iced tea	6	326	**12.5**	**>6**	21	**1457**	>1.5
6 oz. ham tortellini, ½ c. fruit salad, 1 slice sourdough bread, & 12. oz. diet soda*	4	481	**17**	—	**94**	**1040**	<1.5
5 oz. chicken w/barbecue sauce, ½ c. potato salad, & 1 c. sugar-free lemonade	4	354	**15.3**	**3.8**	**137**	**793**	<1.5

* LOSES ADDITIONAL POINTS DUE TO LOW VITAMIN AND MINERAL CONTENT.
NOTE: BOLDFACE NUMBERS INDICATE NUTRITIONAL FACTOR THAT DETRACTS FROM FOOD'S NUTRITIONAL VALUE.

Cafeteria at the Workplace

If you eat at a cafeteria where you work, you are likely to find hot food, as well as cold salads and sandwiches. Keep in mind that you want to eat only the amount of calories that will make you alert and productive in the afternoon. Survey all the possibilities and take advantage of the preview of foods available. Stay away from meat-based entrées in sauces. You probably don't need a hot entrée such as meat loaf and mashed potatoes, an old cafeteria favorite, which is likely to be high in fat even if you tend to eat your biggest meal at lunchtime. You can have more confidence in your choice when you can *see* the "recipe," as in a sandwich or on a salad, rather than with a dish such as escalloped potatoes and ham with all of its "hidden" high-fat ingredients.

CAFETERIA/RESTAURANT LUNCHES	Rating	Calories	Fat (g)	Saturated Fat (g)	Cholesterol (mg)	Sodium (mg)	Fiber (g)
1 c. vegetable soup, ½ turkey sandwich (1 oz. turkey, lettuce, & 1 tsp. mustard), & mineral water	9	233	4	0.6	24	**1094**	>1.5
8 oz. beef teriyaki w/rice & pea pods, 1 c. tea*	8	242	3	—	45	**630**	>1.5
3.5 oz. roasted chicken w/skin, ½ c. mixed vegetables, dinner roll, 1 pat margarine, & iced tea	7	443	**27**	**5.6**	81	366	>1.5
1 c. chili w/beans, 1 piece corn bread, & 1 c. sugar-free lemonade	6	484	**21**	**8**	43	**1132**	>1.5
1 c. New England clam chowder, side salad w/2 tbsp. no oil Italian dressing, & 12 oz. diet soda	5	394	**23**	**12**	83	**1135**	>1.5
1 c. macaroni & cheese, mixed vegetables, & 1 c. coffee	4	467	**23**	**13**	12	30	**<1.5**

* LOSES ADDITIONAL POINTS DUE TO LOW VITAMIN AND MINERAL CONTENT.

NOTE: BOLDFACE NUMBERS INDICATE NUTRITIONAL FACTOR THAT DETRACTS FROM FOOD'S NUTRITIONAL VALUE.

Pack a Lunch from Home

Brown bagging is also coming back into style; 70 percent of those who pack a lunch are, according to the Food and Marketing Institute "Trend Report," adults who work in office settings and choose the timesaving brown-bag alternative over dining out at noon on a regular basis. You've probably noticed the high-tech, insulated lunch pails now on the market. I recently bought a red one called "Ice Man." It contains a dry-ice pack that's kept in the freezer at night and then placed back in the lunch pail when it's in use. Even the six-pack beer coolers make a nice "brown bag."

Brown bagging is my personal favorite. I pack snacks as well as lunch when I'm counseling patients all day. These often include a sandwich or leftovers from the previous night's dinner, such as spaghetti, chicken breast, or pizza. This allows me to accomplish two objectives: I avoid overeating at dinner, and I have a nice treat the next day at lunchtime.

Low-fat cheese and fat-free crackers also transport easily in a brown bag. I've cautioned against adding cheese to protein in a sandwich or other entrée, in order to avoid too much protein, fat, saturated fat, and cholesterol. Cheese can fit into a low-fat diet, however, when it is eaten in *small* amounts as the *sole* source of protein in a lunch. A rule of thumb for cheese and crackers is to slice the cheese thinner than the cracker. More cracker than cheese is a good indication that you are getting more carbohydrate than fat (and fewer calories), exactly what we are aiming for. (See pages 75–76 in Chapter 6 for a complete list of the best crackers and page 77 for the best cheeses.)

And don't forget quantity:

 5 RyKrisp crackers, 1 ounce cheese = 150 calories = 9
15 RyKrisp crackers, 3 ounces cheese = 450 calories = 8
30 RyKrisp crackers, 6 ounces cheese = 900 calories = 7

Many people eat too much cheese on a weekly or even daily basis, particularly those who eat fast, because cheese really is a "fast food." But too much cheese offsets all the other positive changes people have made, from less fatty meat toward more lean meats, grains, and vegetables. Take a look at your diet. If this is true for you, begin to limit the amount of cheese you eat.

If you are willing to carry a brown bag to your office, you'll notice that the menu plans in Chapter 7 make this easy, often suggesting last night's dinner for the next day's lunch. If you are one who has access to a microwave oven at work, use it.

Restaurant Dining

For many, it's rare to have time for a long leisurely lunch, but when you do, whether it's a client meeting or an outing away from the office with co-workers and colleagues, you will be wise to continue the theme of eating sparingly if you want to make the most of your afternoon.

Soups and salads are a good lunch alternative. Trendy restaurants offering an "all you can eat" menu of soup, salad bar, muffins and rolls are often found in roadside shopping malls. The salad bar is a great idea, but you can get too much fat and too many calories here, too. Watch out for those gooey dressings, high-calorie muffins with as much sugar and fat as cake, creamed soups, 25-calorie spoonfuls of vegetables drowning in 150 calories of creamy dressing, and so on. If you choose an item like pasta salad that is heavily "oiled," place a quarter to a half cup on top of your greens and let that be your dressing. Low-calorie salad dressing may be available, or look for a flavorful vinegar, such as a seasoned rice vinegar. Lemon wedges are another alternative.

You may want to choose the hard roll or whole wheat roll instead of the muffins. The muffins are generally quite large and contain a great deal of fat and sugar, canceling out the potential value of the fiber, bran, or fruit that might be in the muffin. Enjoy the flavor of the roll—*without* butter or margarine.

Soups, such as bean, lentil, vegetable, minestrone, won ton, or chicken noodle are nice lunch alternatives. Try a cup rather than a bowl, and choose broth-based rather than *cream* soups, which contain far more fat and calories. If you choose soup in a restaurant, be sure to ask the waiter or waitress about the choices. Can the onion soup be ordered without cheese? Can the black bean soup be served without sour cream? Try a bowl of chili with beans, without added cheese. Is the chowder a tomato-based Manhattan-style (best choice) or a cream-based New England-style? Try to avoid the creamy varieties, and make sure you get adequate calories by adding a slice of bread or a few crackers so that you will not be looking for something else to eat back at the office. Compare these two lunches:

1 cup navy bean with ham **VS.**	1 cup creamy clam chowder
1 whole wheat roll	Blueberry muffin with 1 pat butter
3 cups salad with 1 table-spoon ranch dressing	3 cups salad with 2 table-spoons blue cheese dress-ing
500 calories	1,100 calories
25% fat (14 grams)	50% fat (61 grams)
Rating: 9	Rating: 4

If you prefer to make your lunch meal a hot "dinner"-type selection, stay with lean fish or chicken, then eat lighter in the evening.

The chef salad or cobb salad as entrées may be higher in calories than a sandwich. Beware of too much cheese, bacon, meats, and avocado. A spinach salad may be slightly easier to adapt to healthy guidelines. Ask the waiter or waitress just how the spinach salad is made, then make adjustments. Omit or limit cheese, bacon, and egg, using these fatty foods only to season the salad. Order light dressing or dressing on the side. A whole wheat or sourdough roll is a nice accompaniment. These minor requests make a major difference in the nutritional value of this potentially great lunch:

2 cups spinach	2 cups spinach
1 tablespoon Parmesan cheese	4 tablespoons cheese
1 hard-cooked egg	2 hard-cooked eggs
1 tablespoon crumbled ba-con	3 tablespoons crumbled ba-con

	2 tablespoons dressing 1 hard roll	4 tablespoons dressing 1 hard roll with 1 teaspoon butter
	400 calories 25% fat (11 grams) Rating: 9	900 calories 48% fat (47 grams) Rating: 6

Spinach is high in fiber, iron, and calcium, although some of the calcium is not well absorbed because the oxalic acid in the spinach makes it partially unavailable for absorption in the intestine.

SALADS	Rating	Calories	Fat (g)	Saturated Fat (g)	Cholesterol (mg)	Sodium (mg)	Fiber (g)
Fresh fruit with ½ c. low-fat cottage cheese	10	229	3	1.4	5	468	>1.5
Spinach salad (raw spinach, 2 eggs, tomato, 4 olives, bacon bits, Parmesan cheese, 2 tbsp. olive oil, & pickle)	6	499	**44**	4.7	**555**	**803**	>1.5
Caesar salad (romaine lettuce, egg, tomato, 5 olives, croutons, anchovy, 2 oz. Romano cheese, & 2 tbsp. olive oil)	6	682	**56**	2.2	**332**	**1391**	>1.5
Taco salad (lettuce, tomato, avocado, onion, 2 oz. Cheddar cheese, 1 oz. corn chips, & ⅓ c. chili)	5	607	**40**	**15**	70	**1042**	>1.5
Chef salad (lettuce, tomato, pickle, egg, onion, 2 oz. ham, 2 oz. turkey, 2 oz. beef, 3 oz. cheese, & 2 tbsp. Italian dressing)	4	794	**51**	**23**	**424**	**3360**	>1.5
Cobb salad (lettuce, egg, 2 oz. turkey, tomato, avocado, 2 oz. blue cheese, 3 strips bacon, & 2 tbsp. Italian dressing)	4	678	**54**	**20**	**350**	**2019**	>1.5

NOTE: BOLDFACE NUMBERS INDICATE NUTRITIONAL FACTOR THAT DETRACTS FROM FOOD'S NUTRITIONAL VALUE (see the note on page 22).

We have tried to modify these salads by cutting back on salad dressings, fatty meats, and cheese, which you can do in a restaurant. Be careful about asking for a "vegetarian" salad, since you are likely to get more cheese, which is more fat. Instead, ask for more vegetables, tomatoes and peppers. Pay particular attention to calories, fat, and cholesterol values.

MODIFIED SALADS

	Rating	Calories	Fat (g)	Saturated Fat (g)	Cholesterol (mg)	Sodium (mg)	Fiber (g)
Spinach (spinach, 1 egg, tomato, 2 olives, Parmesan cheese, 1 tbsp. olive oil) & wheat roll	7	342	**24**	2	**278**	542	>1.5
Caesar (romaine lettuce, egg, tomato, 2 olives, croutons, ½ oz. Romano cheese, 1 tbsp. oil) & wheat roll	7	528	**28**	1.8	**288**	543	>1.5
Taco (lettuce, tomato, onion, ½ oz. corn chips, & ¼ c. chili)	7	202	**8**	**2.6**	23	470	>1.5
Chef (lettuce, tomato, pickle, egg, onion, 2 oz. ham, 2 oz. turkey, 2 tbsp. low-cal dressing) & wheat roll	6	364	**13**	4	**318**	**2086**	>1.5
Cobb (lettuce, egg, 2 oz. turkey, 1 oz. blue cheese, 2 tbsp. low-cal dressing) & wheat roll	4	358	**18**	**8**	**350**	**1477**	>1.5

NOTE: BOLDFACE NUMBERS INDICATE NUTRITIONAL FACTOR THAT DETRACTS FROM FOODS NUTRITIONAL VALUE (see the note on page 22).

TIPS ON SANDWICHES

At home, in a brown bag, at a deli, or in a sit-down restaurant, the sandwich is truly fast food. Sandwiches can vary tremendously in fat and calorie content, with some of the old favorites bound to put you over the daily recommended fat intake of 30 percent. What follows are tips on how to get new versions of the old favorites and more, all with less fat and more flavor.

Bread: Whole-grain breads provide more fiber, vitamins, and minerals than white or sourdough bread. Wheat, oat, corn, or rye bread are all good choices (wheat has more fiber than the others, but the other whole grains have more fiber than white bread or rolls). Choose a bagel one day and pita the next—both come as whole grains and are low in sodium. Enjoy a corn or whole wheat tortilla as an alternative. An occasional sourdough roll or white flour tortilla is nice for variety, but plan to eat a whole-grain product at breakfast with cereal, or snack on whole-grain crackers if you have a refined grain at lunch. An open-faced sandwich economizes on calories. My client, Carol, a CPA who often eats lunch at her desk, orders a sandwich from a neighboring deli, eats one half one day and the other half the next.

Meats: Turkey breast is an excellent choice for filling. Although turkey is among the leanest and easiest to order, for the sake of variety and the benefit of extra iron, you may want to select lean beef, ham, or corned beef *once a week*. Choose a Dijon-style mustard instead of mayonnaise. Discard any visible fat on the meat, and limit the amount to *three or four* ounces.

The turkey sandwich described above plus an apple and a cup of low-fat milk will net between 450 and 500 calories. Compare that to a sandwich with six ounces of meat plus cheese and two tablespoons of mayonnaise at a whopping 1,000 calories. The turkey sandwich easily fits into a 1,500-calorie day, and the apple and milk give you needed fiber and calcium as well as fill you up and keep you satisfied.

Processed meats such as bologna, liverwurst, and salami are too high in saturated fat, cholesterol, and sodium. Even processed turkey is salty, so go to a deli or a meat counter that sells turkey fresh roasted, or do your own—it's easy and it's worth the effort.

Vegetarian: Beware of the typical "vegetarian" sandwich. It is usually made with several kinds of cheese, avocado, and mayonnaise, along with lettuce, tomatoes, and perhaps sprouts. This can equal the calories in a Big Mac! If you choose this, limit the amount of cheese, which is high in saturated fat, and have only one slice of the avocado (one-eighth of an avocado, about 40 calories, 35 of which are from fat).

You might try a vegetable sandwich of tomato, lettuce, cucumber, and leftover baked potato. Add a slice of cheese for protein if you like, but avoid adding cheese to meats—it is simply unnecessary to eat that much protein at lunchtime, particularly a higher-fat protein, such as cheese.

Tuna Salad: Premade sandwich fillings, such as tuna salad or even chicken or egg, are not as "safe" as lean, unembellished slices of turkey, chicken, beef, or ham, and therefore are not an ideal daily choice, unless you make your own. These fillings are usually made with a substantial amount of mayonnaise, and have a very high fat content.

When the tuna salad is displayed in a case where you can see it, check to see how much mayonnaise is in the mixture. If you are in a restaurant, ask your waitress or waiter. They will often be quite candid. If you decide to order the tuna salad, simply say: "Could I have a tuna salad sandwich on wheat bread, with lettuce and tomatoes, but no extra mayonnaise on the bread, and less than the usual amount of tuna, about a quarter to a half cup." Or, it is a perfectly acceptable solution to get the full sandwich of three quarters to one cup of tuna salad and then remove half of it from between the two slices of bread. Better to waste it than add it to your waist.

At home, of course, use a small amount of the reduced fat mayonnaise or better yet, use low-fat yogurt. A combination of the two works well. See my recipe for Tuna Salad on Whole Wheat in Chapter 11, which suggests the addition of vegetables (onions, celery, carrots, et cetera) to dilute fat calories and increase fiber. The recipe shows a comparison of my sandwich to the typical tuna salad sandwich. The nutritional impact of using less fat and more vegetables is impressive.

Add-ons: Hold the mayonnaise, or go easy on it. Use the lower-calorie light mayonnaise, which contains one-third less calories. Put it on and then scrape it off or try the salad spray by Richard Simmons. Add vegetables, such as lettuce and tomato, that help to keep the sandwich moist. Ketchup and mustard are low-fat, high-flavor condiments at 15 calories per tablespoon. They contribute about 150 milligrams of sodium per tablespoon, so don't go overboard. If sodium is a concern, try horseradish: it's half the calories and one-tenth the sodium.

Have a standard sandwich—one that meets *your standards*. Get in the habit of asking first for what you *do* want on the sandwich, rather than what you *don't* want on it. Be specific, for example: *three to four ounces* of *lean* meat, poultry or fish, on *whole-grain* bread, with mustard, lettuce and tomato. This choice meets the nutritional criteria of adequate, not excessive, protein, moderate carbohydrate, and it's low in fat.

A PROBLEM

For those who are at home during the day, either with children or perhaps working out of their home, access to food can be a challenge, requiring particular structure. If you are stuck in the "grazing" habit with a steady stream of snacking that has you eating too many calories and in a weight-gain mode, make a change. Introduce *structure* to your day. Plan activities that include *specific* times for eating and exercising. Here is the place to use the time-tested behavior-modification technique of eating only in *one* place. Designate this spot with a formal table setting: place mat, napkin, and so on. Clean up when you are finished. Get involved with activities other than food that demand your attention and provide you with stimulation. Volunteer to feed the homeless, enroll in a class, or go to the library to read. Take care of both your physical and psychological needs. A balanced life is one of the most important keys to normal weight and good health.

Whether you work at home or not, structured *routine* can support positive lifestyle changes. Many people insist they do not have a routine, but once they actually look at what they eat on a one- or two-week basis, it is apparent that a routine emerges. Make it a *good* routine that supports your goals. Good choices will become automatic by practicing them.

SANDWICHES

	Rating	Calories	Fat (g)	Saturated Fat (g)	Cholesterol (mg)	Sodium (mg)	Fiber (g)
2 oz. turkey breast on wheat toast w/romaine lettuce, tomato slice, & 1 tsp. mustard	10	343	5.0	2.5	65	288	>1.5
3 oz. low-sodium water-packed tuna, 1 tbsp. lite mayo, romaine lettuce, & 2 slices wheat bread	10	244	4	0.6	24	442	>1.5
3 oz. lean roast beef, ¼ c. cabbage, 1 tsp. mustard, & 2 slices rye bread	9	269	5.6	1.5	39	**1065**	>1.5
2 slices lean ham, bell pepper, alfalfa sprouts, 1 tsp. mustard in pita pocket	9	187	3	1	30	**1219**	>1.5
3 oz. corned beef, sauerkraut, 1 tsp. mustard, & 1 oz. lite Swiss cheese on 2 slices rye bread	9	236	6	2.8	42	**1330**	>1.5
Bagel w/lox, 1 tsp. cream cheese, & onion	9	300	8	2.2	28	**950**	>1.5
Egg salad (1 egg, 1 tbsp. lite mayo, diced celery, & watercress) on a bagel	8	275	**10**	2.2	**278**	375	>1.5
1 tbsp. peanut butter, 1 tsp. jelly, & 2 slices white bread	8	185	**11.5**	1.7	0	380	>1.5
Club (white toast, 2 oz. turkey, 2 oz. ham, 2 oz. lite Swiss cheese, 1 tbsp. lite mayo)	7	449	**16.5**	**6**	72	**2598**	>1.5
Vegetarian (2 slices wheat bread, ¼ avocado, 2 oz. lite Swiss cheese, 1 tbsp. lite mayo, tomato, onion, bell pepper, cucumber & carrot)	6	422	**18**	**5.6**	28	**1100**	>1.5
Italian sub (roll, mortadella, salami, bologna, provolone cheese, 1 tbsp. lite mayo, tomato, & onion)	4	741	**35**	**11.6**	56	**1941**	**<1.5**
3 oz. pastrami, 2 slices rye bread, 1 tsp. mustard, 1 tbsp. lite mayo, romaine lettuce, tomato, & onion*	4	506	**30**	**9.5**	82	**1508**	>1.5

* LOSES ADDITIONAL POINTS DUE TO LOW VITAMIN AND MINERAL CONTENT.

NOTE: BOLDFACE NUMBERS INDICATE NUTRITIONAL FACTOR THAT DETRACTS FROM FOOD'S NUTRITIONAL VALUE (see the note on page 22).

ALL LUNCHES

	Rating	Calories	Fat (g)	Saturated Fat (g)	Cholesterol (mg)	Sodium (mg)	Fiber (g)
McDonald's Chunky Chicken Salad w/1 tbsp. Lite Vinaigrette Dressing	10	140	3.4	0.9	78	230	>1.5
Turkey on wheat bread	10	343	5.0	2.5	65	288	>1.5
Low-fat tuna salad on wheat bread	10	244	4	0.6	24	442	>1.5
Fresh fruit salad w/low-fat cottage cheese	10	229	3	1.4	5	468	>1.5
Vegetable soup & ½ turkey sandwich	9	233	4	0.6	24	**1094**	>1.5
Plain baked potato & salad w/low-cal dressing	9	397	7	<5	0	**315**	>1.5
Wendy's Chili and plain baked potato	9	490	7	2.6	45	**750**	>1.5
Lean roast beef on rye	9	269	5.6	1.5	39	**1065**	>1.5

	Rating	Calories	Fat (g)	Saturated Fat (g)	Cholesterol (mg)	Sodium (mg)	Fiber (g)
Lean ham in pita	9	187	3	1	30	**1219**	>1.5
Bagel w/lox & cream cheese	9	300	8	2.2	28	**950**	>1.5
Corned beef & Swiss in pita	9	236	6	2.8	42	**1330**	>1.5
2 slices cheese pizza	9	376	10	**5.5**	19	484	6.4
Bean burrito	9	357	10	2.9	9	**888**	>1.5
Roast beef sandwich & salad w/low-cal dressing	8	533	13.5	—	60	**1290**	>1.5
Chicken fajita pita	8	292	8	2.9	34	**704**	<1.5
Peanut butter & jelly on wheat bread	8	185	**11.5**	1.7	0	380	>1.5
Broccoli & cheese stuffed potato	8	400	**16**	2.9	<15	455	>1.5
Egg salad on a bagel	8	275	**10**	2.2	**278**	375	>1.5
Crab salad, wheat roll & low-fat yogurt	8	295	9	**4**	65	344	>1.5
Rigatoni w/ham & peas	8	350	9	—	50	**1376**	>1.5
Beef teriyaki w/rice & pea pods	8	242	3	—	45	**630**	>1.5
Taco salad w/corn chips & chili	7	202	**8**	**2.6**	23	470	>1.5
Club on white bread	7	490	**16.5**	**6**	72	**2597**	<1.5
Spinach salad w/1 egg, roll, & 1 tbsp. olive oil	7	342	**24**	2	**278**	542	>1.5
Roasted chicken, vegetables, & roll w/margarine	7	443	**27**	**5.6**	81	366	>1.5
Extra crispy drumstick, corn & potatoes	7	408	**15**	4	65	584	**<1.5**
Caesar salad w/1 egg, cheese, roll & 1 tbsp. oil	7	528	**28**	1.8	**288**	543	>1.5
Vegetarian on wheat bread	6	422	**18**	**5.6**	28	**1100**	>1.5
Spinach salad w/2 eggs & 2 tbsp. olive oil	6	499	**44**	4.7	**555**	803	>1.5
Lasagna & green salad	6	326	**12.5**	**>6**	21	**1457**	>1.5
Chili & corn bread	6	484	**21**	**8**	43	**1132**	>1.5
Chef salad w/egg, ham, turkey, roll, & 1 tbsp. dressing	6	364	**13**	4	**318**	**2086**	>1.5
Caesar salad w/egg, anchovy, cheese, & 2 tbsp. oil	6	682	**56**	2.2	**332**	**1391**	>1.5
Plain hamburger & frozen yogurt cone	6	360	10.3	**4**	40	580	**<1.5**
Clam chowder, side salad w/o dressing	5	394	**23**	**12**	83	**1135**	>1.5
Taco salad w/avocado, cheese, chips, & chili	5	607	**40**	**15**	70	**1042**	>1.5
Plain hamburger & salad w/low-cal dressing	5	350	**13.8**	**5.3**	78	**735**	**<1.5**
Pastrami on rye	4	506	**30**	**9.5**	82	**1508**	>1.5
Macaroni & cheese & mixed vegetables	4	467	**23**	**13**	12	30	**<1.5**
Italian submarine on roll	4	741	**35**	**11.6**	56	**1941**	**<1.5**
Ham tortellini, salad & bread	4	481	**17**	—	**94**	**1040**	**<1.5**
Cobb salad w/egg, turkey, cheese & 2 tbsp. dressing	4	678	**54**	**20**	**350**	**2019**	>1.5
Chef salad w/ham, turkey, beef, cheese, & oil	4	794	**51**	**23**	**424**	**3360**	>1.5
Barbecue chicken, potato salad	4	354	**15.3**	3.8	**137**	**793**	**<1.5**
Whopper & regular french fries	2	955	**56**	**22**	**111**	**1106**	**<1.5**

NOTE: BOLDFACE NUMBERS INDICATE NUTRITIONAL FACTOR THAT DETRACTS FROM FOOD'S NUTRITIONAL VALUE (see the note on page 22).

CHAPTER · 5

THE FAST-FOOD DINNER

THE NEW AMERICAN DINNER

Dinner is a meal often eaten at home, even by busy people. In fact, "eating in" is the newest trend in dinner. Perhaps Americans recognize something special about spending more time at home with their family. Of course, for some, home is simply the place to eat and run again. Perhaps we choose the privacy of our home as a retreat after a hard day in a hectic work environment. Whatever the reason, it's a fact that many of us are returning to our very own kitchens at dinnertime. Some say this indicates a return to the basic values of the fifties.

But there's a difference. Today, the maximum time we want to spend cooking a meal is thirty minutes—and that's stretching it for many of us. We may not want to "cook" at all. We are more likely to pick up some of our dinner on our way home, or call out for a special delivery pizza or reheat a low-calorie, "gourmet" frozen entrée.

To further complicate matters, our palates have also come of age. We not only want convenience food, we also expect quality. And that means quality in terms of taste and nutritional value. We want fast food, but we don't want to go to the corner hamburger stand. And the food industry knows it. Food manufacturers and supermarkets are attempting to meet our needs with new convenience products, fresh pasta, salad bars, cooked meats, frozen dinners, and snacks. Even take-out meals are now available at many supermarkets. What follows is a review of dinner options including carry-out, frozen, and meals you are likely to prepare at home.

DELIS

The deli can offer a supplemental salad or side dish to a home-cooked meal, or it can offer the entrée itself: a marinated chicken, a lamb or beef brochette, a stuffed pork chop, et cetera. No real cooking is necessary—just follow simple instructions to bake, broil, or barbecue. Or you can buy a pasta dish that merely needs to be heated in the microwave oven. Delis appeal to our desire for convenience, as well as for fresh, flavorful "home" cooking. Deli fare increasingly reflects our interest in reducing fat and cholesterol. New lines of deli products with lighter and less sauce are available. Check our ratings for deli foods in Chapter 8.

As you do your deli shopping, follow the 1-to-5 rule. That's a ratio calling for approximately 1 part animal protein for every 5 parts vegetable or starch: for example, a marinated chicken (a four-ounce portion per person, about one breast) supplemented with two cups of salad, vegetable, rice, or potato. The amount of starch and vegetable depends on your calorie need, and should be adjusted accordingly! Remember vegetables are 20–30 calories per cup, and starches are generally 160 calories per cup. See portion sizes on fast-food diet menu plans, pages 89–109, for examples. The easiest way to calculate it is to simply look at the plate. Try a beef or lamb kabob and vegetable where you have built-in portion control. When this choice is supplemented with salad or rice, you can achieve a 1-to-5 ratio quite easily.

Choose a tomato sauce which is likely to contain olive oil instead of a cream-based sauce which contains butterfat from cream. Olive oil is monounsaturated, as opposed to a cream-based sauce, which is a more saturated fat with cholesterol.

SPAGHETTI DINNERS	Rating	Calories	Fat (g)	Saturated Fat (g)	Cholesterol (mg)	Sodium (mg)	Fiber (g)
1½ c. spaghetti w/ ⅓ c. bottled sauce (Prego), salad, 2 tbsp. Italian dressing, & garlic toast w/margarine	7	637	**26**	5	1	**926**	>1.5
Same as above with 2 oz. lean ground beef	6	797	**37**	9	50	**971**	>1.5
Same as first, except alfredo cream sauce instead of tomato sauce	4	834	**50.4**	**22**	94	**884**	>1.5

NOTE: BOLDFACE NUMBERS INDICATE NUTRITIONAL FACTOR THAT DETRACTS FROM FOOD'S NUTRITIONAL VALUE (see the note on page 22).

Supermarkets and their deli sections, in particular, are being promoted as the new alternative to the singles bar in some locales. There is a Lucky supermarket, for example, across from a popular fitness gym in the San Diego area where the scene gets hot between 5:00 and 7:00 P.M. Single men and women just finished with their workday, or their workout, sling a red plastic shopping basket on their arm, quietly hum along to the latest rock 'n' roll song playing overhead, and set out to buy their dinner. They pick out a ready-made salad at the salad bar or a head of lettuce in the produce section, then pick up a fresh pasta and a gourmet sauce at the deli, then pass by the bakery department for a loaf of hot fresh French bread—maybe even already buttered and seasoned for garlic toast.

One Safeway store in San Rafael, California, offers serious competition to Chinese take-out restaurants! It has hired its own Chinese chef. You can do one-stop shopping, get your stir-fry and your carton of low-fat milk for the morning breakfast and any other items you need.

TAKE-OUT

A simple call or visit to a restaurant that offers food to go can feed your dinner hunger and be satisfying. Be choosy in your selection, though, and pass by fatty fried foods such as fried chicken or fish, and french fries. Try picking up Chinese food, ordering a pizza or Mexican food.

Chinese Food

Choose dishes that feature a vegetable along with a protein, to increase vitamin-mineral content, fiber, and decrease fat and cholesterol. Steer away from the ones with cashews and peanuts rather than vegetables. Order steamed rice. Once you have ordered the right food, be careful to limit the amount you eat.

CHINESE DINNERS

	Rating	Calories	Fat (g)	Saturated Fat (g)	Cholesterol (mg)	Sodium (mg)	Fiber (g)
Stir-fried chicken w/vegetables (½ skinless chicken breast, ½ c. steamed rice, 1 stalk celery, ¼ c. green pepper, ½ hot red pepper, ⅓ carrot, ⅓ c. chopped mushrooms, 1 tbsp. oil, 1 tsp. soy sauce & cornstarch)	9	439	**17**	3.2	73	315	>1.5
Shrimp w/pea pods (4 oz. shrimp, 2 oz. pea pods, 1 tbsp. oil, ½ c. steamed rice, & 1 oz. wine)	8	386	**14.5**	2.6	**221**	256	>1.5
Beef w/broccoli (3.5 oz. beef, ¼ c. broccoli, ½ c. steamed rice, 1 tbsp. oil, & 1 tbsp. soy sauce)	6	459	**23**	**5.9**	84	**888**	>1.5
Sweet & sour pork (3.5 oz. pork, 1 tsp. soy sauce, 3 tbsp. cornstarch, ¼ c. onion, ¼ c. pineapple, ½ bell pepper, 1.5 tbsp. sugar, 1 tbsp. ketchup, 2 tbsp. oil, & ½ c. steamed rice)*	4	732	**32.4**	6.3	93	362	<1.5

* LOSES ADDITIONAL POINTS DUE TO HIGH SUGAR AND LOW VITAMIN AND MINERAL CONTENT.
NOTE: BOLDFACE NUMBERS INDICATE NUTRITIONAL FACTOR THAT DETRACTS FROM FOOD'S NUTRITIONAL VALUE (see the note on page 22).

Pizza

Always eat a salad *before* you eat the pizza, particularly if you are really hungry. It can make the difference between eating two or three more pieces than you might eat if you skipped the salad. It also increases fiber, vitamins, and minerals. If you choose "meat pizza," pepperoni or Canadian bacon is a better choice than sausage or hamburger. Order *vegetarian* pizza (bell peppers, onions, mushrooms, tomato slices) with *light* cheese. Never order "extra" cheese. You will learn not to miss the high-fat smoked meats. Just let go of old habits and replace them with something that will get you what you want in the long term.

PIZZA DINNERS* 1 slice = ⅛ of 14″ pizza

	Rating	Calories	Fat (g)	Saturated Fat (g)	Cholesterol (mg)	Sodium (mg)	Fiber (g)
1 slice vegetarian pizza (1 oz. cheese, mushrooms, 1 olive, green peppers, onion, 2 oz. tomatoes)	7	303	**11**	**5.5**	22	599	>4
2 slices vegetarian pizza (2 oz. cheese, ⅓ oz. mushrooms, 3 olives, ½ oz. green peppers, 1 oz. onion, 4 oz. tomatoes)	6	606	**22**	**11**	44	**1199**	>8
2 slices vegetarian w/double cheese	5	768	**34**	**18**	88	**1414**	>10
2 slices deluxe pizza (6 oz. cheese, 1 oz. sausage, 3 oz. pepperoni, ⅓ oz. green peppers, ¼ oz. mushrooms, 3 olives, ¾ oz. onion, 3 oz. tomatoes)	4	1055	**61.2**	**27**	194	**2585**	>10

* ADDING SALAD AND GARLIC BREAD TO A PIZZA DINNER WILL ADD VITAMINS A AND C AS WELL AS INCREASING COMPLEX CARBOHYDRATES AND FIBER.
NOTE: BOLDFACE NUMBERS INDICATE NUTRITIONAL FACTOR THAT DETRACTS FROM FOOD'S NUTRITIONAL VALUE (see the note on page 22).

Mexican

Order *à la carte*. A single item will probably satisfy your hunger, the fajita or a burrito. Again, try to add a salad to your meal, if possible. Beware of tostadas, which emphasize cheese, meat, avocado, and sour cream over salad greens—real high-fat hazards.

MEXICAN DINNERS	Rating	Calories	Fat (g)	Saturated Fat (g)	Cholesterol (mg)	Sodium (mg)	Fiber (g)
Chicken fajita (3 oz. chicken, bell peppers, corn tortilla, onion, 1 tbsp. oil, ½ c. rice, ½ c. beans)	9	542	16.2	3.5	73	**662**	>1.5
Chicken burrito (flour tortilla, 4 oz. chicken, onion, green chilies, 15 chips, ¼ c. salsa), side salad & 1 tbsp. oil & vinegar dressing	7	615	**24.5**	5	87	**1273**	>1.5
Chicken enchiladas (2 corn tortillas, 3 oz. chicken, 2 oz. sauce, 2 oz. cheese, 15 chips, ¼ c. salsa) side salad & 1 tbsp. dressing	4	691	**42**	**17**	**133**	**1244**	>1.5
Deluxe nachos (2 oz. tortilla chips, 2 oz. Cheddar cheese sauce, ¾ c. refried beans, 2 oz. ground beef, ¼ tomato, ¼ c. jalapeño peppers, 3 tbsp. sour cream, 3 tbsp. guacamole, & 6 medium chopped olives)	4	980	**55.5**	**20**	77	**1941**	**<1.5**
Carne asada burrito (flour tortilla, 4 oz. roast beef, green chilies, 15 chips, ¼ c. salsa, 1 tbsp. oil, 3 tbsp. sour cream, & 3 tbsp. guacamole), ½ c. rice, ½ c. refried beans	3	1297	**76.2**	**23.4**	**135**	**1928**	**<1.5**

NOTE: BOLDFACE NUMBERS INDICATE NUTRITIONAL FACTOR THAT DETRACTS FROM FOOD'S NUTRITIONAL VALUE (see the note on page 22).

Chicken

This has become a popular carry-out dinner as chicken continues to gain in public favor over beef. But be aware that the nutritional advantages of chicken are diminished as the spit-roasted chicken is cooked in its skin, increasing fat content. You may notice that it's a lot greasier than your own chicken, which has had the skin removed before cooking. Again, eat only one or two pieces instead of three or four, and balance the meal with rice or potato, vegetable or salad.

CHICKEN DINNERS

	Rating	Calories	Fat (g)	Saturated Fat (g)	Cholesterol (mg)	Sodium (mg)	Fiber (g)
½ skinless chicken breast, baked potato, 2 tbsp. lite sour cream, salad, & 2 tbsp. low-cal dressing	9	485	13	**5.6**	88	411	>1.5
½ roasted chicken breast w/skin, ½ c. rice, salad & 1 tbsp. vinegar & oil dressing	7	428	**18.7**	**6.2**	84	153	>1.5
Kentucky Fried Chicken Original Recipe side breast, coleslaw, mashed potatoes, & gravy*	5	457	**24.7**	**5.7**	82	**1274**	>1.5
McDonald's McChicken Sandwich*	5	490	**28.6**	5.4	43	**780**	<1.5
McDonald's Chicken McNuggets w/sweet & sour sauce, side salad, & ½ packet (2 tbsp.) lite vinaigrette dressing	4	440	**20.8**	**5.7**	106	**945**	<1.5

* LOSES ADDITIONAL POINTS DUE TO LOW VITAMIN AND MINERAL CONTENT.
NOTE: BOLDFACE NUMBERS INDICATE NUTRITIONAL FACTOR THAT DETRACTS FROM FOOD'S NUTRITIONAL VALUE (see the note on page 22).

The key to take-out dining success is to know *where* you'd like to order out—*ahead of time.* Take a moment now to make a list of the restaurants that are in your neighborhood, on the way home from work, or near your home. Look up their phone numbers and record them in your address book or weekly planner. Choose the places that are willing to honor any special requests that you might have, the requests that will ensure that you do not compromise your nutritional objectives.

COOKING AT HOME

Those precious few meals that are actually prepared at home can now be far less labor-intensive. Fewer items are made from scratch and fewer are served per meal. Take what you know about low-fat cooking and redistribute the mainstays of Mom's square meals. Meat becomes a "seasoning" mixed with vegetables in a soup, stew, or stir-fry. These meals are easily served in a single pot, rather than as a multicourse dinner. A salad may accompany the meal, but generally only one or two items are served per meal. Meats can be used to add flavor rather than serve as a main dish. This helps to limit calories, fat, and cholesterol.

Even if you do prepare Mom's old standbys of meat, potato, and vegetable, give it a leaner look. Go for the leaner cuts of meat and serve smaller portions. Choose lean animal protein such as chicken, fish, or lean red meat—broiled, baked or barbecued—not fried.

FISH DINNERS

	Rating	Calories	Fat (g)	Saturated Fat (g)	Cholesterol (mg)	Sodium (mg)	Fiber (g)
6 oz. baked or broiled halibut, ½ tsp. oil, baked potato w/1 tsp. margarine, salad, & 1 tbsp. low-cal dressing	10	563	13.6	2.3	73	406	>1.5
6 oz. baked or broiled sole, ½ tsp. oil, baked potato w/1 tsp. margarine, salad & 1 tbsp. low-cal dressing	10	440	10.1	1.5	84	531	>1.5
Same as above except shrimp instead of sole	8	489	10	1.9	**332**	**668**	>1.5
Long John Silver's 3-Piece Fish Dinner (3 fish, fryes, slaw, & 2 hushpuppies)*	5	960	**44**	10	**100**	**1890**	>1.5

* LOSES ADDITIONAL POINTS DUE TO LOW VITAMIN AND MINERAL CONTENT.

NOTE: BOLDFACE NUMBERS INDICATE NUTRITIONAL FACTOR THAT DETRACTS FROM FOOD'S NUTRITIONAL VALUE (see the note on page 22).

Allow larger servings of vegetables to replace smaller servings of meat. This automatically increases fiber and complex carbohydrate, and that's what we're after. Take another step in the revolutionary eating process as you limit fats *added* to salads, pastas, potatoes, and bread.

For more excitement at home, get into ethnic cuisine—Mexican, Japanese, Chinese, Mediterranean. You'll find a number of ideas to help you out in Chapter 14, "Main Dishes."

The sauces and marinades in my recipe collection, Part II, will give you flavor without fat. If you choose beef, pork, or veal, remember that the leanest cuts are from the leg or loin, called round or tenderloin. The rule of thumb when cooking these tender cuts of meat is "hot and fast," great for a stir-fry or a barbecue. For less tender cuts, it's best to add a fat-free liquid (water, broth, or wine) and "braise" or stew for longer periods of time. Do remember that the fat content of lean beef can be almost as low as chicken, but that it is slightly higher in saturated fats, so try to hold beef intake to once a week.

RED MEAT DINNERS

	Rating	Calories	Fat (g)	Saturated Fat (g)	Cholesterol (mg)	Sodium (mg)	Fiber (g)
3 oz. lean sirloin beef, baked potato, 1 tsp. margarine, & salad w/2 tsp. low-cal dressing	8	514	**21.8**	2.9	78	494	>1.5
Same as above with 3 oz. lean, roasted pork loin	8	543	**26.4**	4.1	79	497	>1.5
Same as above with 6 oz. beef	7	691	**29.2**	6	**154**	550	>1.5
Same as above with 9 oz. beef	6	868	**36.4**	9.1	**230**	**606**	>1.5

NOTE: BOLDFACE NUMBERS INDICATE NUTRITIONAL FACTOR THAT DETRACTS FROM FOOD'S NUTRITIONAL VALUE (see the note on page 22).

Rotational Meals

People tend to eat the same right foods all the time, or the same *wrong* foods all the time, especially at dinner. Do you tend to rotate through the same repertoire of meals on a regular basis? This is fine—if the meals provide a good balance. Check the charts to determine your balance.

A caution to women. The growing trend toward eliminating red meat altogether has been paralleled by an increase in anemia among women, particularly among young women who are restricting their calories in an attempt to lose weight. Consequently, they feel tired and fatigued and may be suffering from low iron. Beef is a good source of iron, and lean meat once a week, without added fats or french fries and desserts, could be helpful to prevent this all-too-common scenario.

Microwave ovens are great for leftovers. No mess, no fuss, just reheat without overcooking. Whether it's a doggie bag from the restaurant or pasta from last night's dinner, it's easy to make a second meal that may even be more appreciated than the first. Mix leftovers with other foods. Perhaps rice can be lightly stir-fried with vegetables, or last night's baked potato can be cut into strips and light steamed or broiled into a French fry. It's often a good idea to add one fresh food to the leftovers, ideally a salad or a freshly steamed vegetable, such as carrots or asparagus, or green beans—just enough to make this dinner a little bit different from its origins.

BEYOND FROZEN DINNERS

According to Mona Doyle, food trend analyst and president of the Consumer Network in Philadelphia, microwave ovens are contributing significantly to dietary changes. Her studies show that 75 to 80 percent of all U.S. households have them and 90 percent of homes are projected to have them by the year 2000. Microwavable products are up in sales 64 percent from 1986 to 1988, including not only frozen dinners, but bite-size and one-hand eating foods that fit into our fast lives. These include egg rolls, mini-tacos, and French bread pizza. They can be hot snacks, appetizers, or small meals. Many frozen products are popular with children, 40 percent of whom assist in preparing their own meals. That means children may prepare anything from frozen dinners in the oven to sandwiches to cookies from Tollhouse cookie dough. In fact, Con Agra has a new frozen product that caters exclusively to children called Kid's Cuisine, meals that actually meet our 30 percent fat guidelines for healthy eating. Here is a list of ten frozen dinners and their varying ranges of ratings.

TEN FROZEN DINNERS	Rating	Calories	Fat (g)	Saturated Fat (g)	Cholesterol (mg)	Sodium (mg)	Fiber (g)
Healthy Choice breast of turkey dinner*	9	270	5	2	55	469	>1.5
Healthy Choice chicken Oriental dinner*	9	210	1	<1	45	410	>1.5
Stouffers Right Course vegetarian chili with seasoned rice*	9	280	7	1	0	590	>1.5
The Budget Gourmet Light Mandarin chicken*	8	300	6	<3	<90	**690**	>1.5
Light & Elegant Florentine lasagna	8	280	5	<3	25	**980**	<1.5
Le Menu Light Style Swedish meatballs	7	260	8	**3**	40	**700**	<1.5
Banquet fried chicken	7	359	11	<6	<90	**1831**	<1.5
Pillsbury Cheese French bread pizza*	5	339	**13.5**	>6	<90	574	>1.5
¼ Celeste Deluxe pizza*	4	378	**22**	>6	<90	**953**	>1.5
Banquet macaroni & cheese*	3	344	**17**	>6	<90	**930**	<1.5

* LOSES ADDITIONAL POINTS DUE TO LOW VITAMIN AND MINERAL CONTENT.

NOTE: BOLDFACE NUMBERS INDICATE NUTRITIONAL FACTOR THAT DETRACTS FROM FOOD'S NUTRITIONAL VALUE (see the note on page 22).

If you have quit buying vegetables because they spoil in the crisper before you have a chance to eat them, there are new single-serving microwave broccoli, green beans, and mixed vegetables. As you probably know, vegetables are one of the first foods to go when we eat in a hurry. These new products, along with the microwave technology, make it easy to eat not only fast, but healthy, too. (See Chapter 8 for ratings of all the major frozen-food offerings.)

ALL DINNERS	Rating	Calories	Fat (g)	Saturated Fat (g)	Cholesterol (mg)	Sodium (mg)	Fiber (g)
Halibut	10	563	**13.6**	2.3	73	406	>1.5
Sole	10	440	**10.1**	1.5	**84**	531	>1.5
Chicken fajita	9	542	**16.2**	3.5	73	**662**	>1.5
Stir-fried chicken with vegetables	9	439	**17**	3.2	73	315	>1.5
½ skinless chicken breast	9	485	**13**	5.6	88	411	>1.5
Shrimp with pea pods	8	386	**14.5**	2.6	**221**	256	>1.5
Shrimp	8	489	**10**	1.9	**332**	**668**	>1.5
3 oz. lean sirloin beef	8	514	**21.8**	2.9	78	494	>1.5
3 oz. pork loin	8	543	**26.4**	4.1	79	497	>1.5
6 oz. lean sirloin beef	7	691	**29.2**	6	**154**	550	>1.5
Spaghetti with tomato sauce	7	637	**26**	5	1	**926**	>1.5
½ roasted chicken breast	7	428	**18.7**	6.2	84	153	>1.5
1 slice vegetarian pizza	7	303	**11**	5.5	22	599	>4
Chicken burrito	7	615	**24.5**	5	87	**1273**	>1.5
9 oz. lean sirloin beef	6	868	**36.4**	9.1	**230**	606	>1.5
Beef with broccoli	6	459	**23**	5.9	84	**888**	>1.5
Spaghetti with meat sauce	6	797	**37**	**9**	50	971	>1.5
2 slices vegetarian pizza	6	606	**22**	**11**	44	**1199**	>8
Kentucky Fried Chicken	5	457	**24.7**	**5.7**	82	**1274**	>1.5
2 slices vegetarian pizza w/double cheese	5	768	**34**	**18**	88	**1414**	>10
Long John Silver's Fish Dinner	5	960	**44**	10	**100**	**1890**	>1.5
McDonald's McChicken Sandwich	5	490	**28.6**	5.4	43	**780**	<1.5
Sweet & sour pork	4	732	**32.4**	6.3	**93**	362	<1.5
McDonald's Chicken McNuggets Dinner	4	440	**20.8**	**5.7**	106	**945**	<1.5
Chicken enchiladas	4	691	**42**	**17**	133	**1244**	>1.5
Spaghetti w/alfredo sauce	4	834	**50.4**	22	**94**	**884**	>1.5
Deluxe nachos	4	980	**55.5**	20	77	**1941**	<1.5
2 slices deluxe pizza	4	1055	**61.2**	27	**194**	**2585**	>10
Carne asada burrito	3	1297	**76.2**	**23.4**	135	**1928**	<1.5

NOTE: BOLDFACE NUMBERS INDICATE NUTRITIONAL FACTOR THAT DETRACTS FROM FOOD'S NUTRITIONAL VALUE (see the note on page 22).

CHAPTER · 6

FAST-FOOD SNACKS, DESSERTS, AND BEVERAGES

SNACKING

The issue of snacking confuses people. Is it a good habit or a bad one? Most assume that it's bad. It isn't—not if you choose wisely and use some restraint. These between-meal snacks can actually be beneficial; here's why.

Weight Management

Used properly, snacking can cut down on the size of meals, particularly lunch and dinner, and in this way, help control weight. Snacking can help prevent too great a calorie deficit during dieting, and thus control hunger. I advise dieting clients to have yogurt, fruit, or low-fat crackers between meals. The idea, of course, is not to fill up, but to snack just enough so that by lunch or dinner time you will be in control of your choices, instead of being swayed by a rumbling stomach. Keep snacks light so that snack-plus-meal does not lead to sluggishness and calorie overload. The day's snacks should equal *25 percent* of your total daily caloric intake; the remaining 75 percent is derived from breakfast, lunch, and dinner; so, if you need 1,600 calories a day, you should get about 400 calories from snacks.

Nutrition Boost

Snacking can help boost the vitamin, mineral, and fiber content of your diet. This is especially important for growing children, who pound per pound, require as much iron and calcium as a thirty-year-old man who weighs 150 pounds. They require even more protein, thiamin, riboflavin, niacin, and vitamins B-6 and B-12. This means the calories a child consumes need to be chosen with particular care so that they provide good sources of nutrients along with calories. I recently saw a seven-year-old boy named Nicky whose well-intentioned mother limited snacks she considered "bad." She insisted, for example, that he snack on sugar-free Popsicles rather than on pudding pops made from milk. She put his peanut butter on celery sticks instead of bread. But the boy was underweight. These are good snacks, but this boy is a special case. He needed snacks to provide extra calories and nutrients.

Small women who have relatively low calorie requirements, say 1,200, yet still need 800 milligrams of calcium, 12 milligrams of zinc, and 180 micrograms of folic acid per day, may also have a special need of snacking.

Fat Storage

Snacking in-between meals may also improve the way our bodies store fat. As mentioned in the lunch chapter, those who eat more frequently throughout the day tend to store less body fat than those who consume most or all of their calories at one or two feedings.

The message is to eat the *right* snacks, and you'll meet the needs for calories and good health. Choose appropriate snacks that control hunger and satisfy your appetite. The Fast-Food Diet is designed to be an eating style you will stay with for the long term. Therefore, snacking must be built in. By using our food guide and checking the ratings of your selections, you can judge snacks and choose those with the best nutritional and caloric value. You may find an 8, 9 or 10 snack that you enjoy as much as a 1, 2, or 3, so why not switch? Here is a list of a few snacks along with their fast-food rating.

Rating of Selected Snacks

Cookies:	Rating
Fig bars and gingersnaps	6
Vanilla wafers	4
Pepperidge Farm varieties	2

Fruits:	
Mango	10
Banana	9
Apple	8

Vegetables:	
Broccoli	10
Cucumber & celery	7

Crackers and Chips:	
Rye wafers	8
Triscuits	6
Saltines	6
Potato chips	3

Nuts/Seeds:	Rating
Sesame seeds	6
Peanuts	4
Macadamia nuts	3

Granola Bars:	
Smart Start Bars	5
Rice Krispies bars	5
Figurines and Breakfast Bars	4
New Trail bars	2

Dips and Spreads:	
Refried beans	8
Peanut butter	4
Sour cream	2

Bread:	
Whole grain	8
White	7

Learn to read labels. Pay attention to the list of ingredients. They are listed in descending order of amount by weight. In other words, the first ingredient is present in the largest amount, and the last ingredient in the smallest amount.

THE FAST-FOOD SNACKING SYSTEM

When to Snack and When Not to Snack

"Snack only when you are hungry." That's easy advice to give. It's also good advice. We get into trouble when we ignore signals from our stomachs and brains—signals of either hunger or satiety. Learn to listen to the body and respond appropriately.

Of course, for some the signals get distorted; in a minority of people the signals never quit screaming, "Eat!" In those people, snacking becomes compulsive. Food in these cases becomes addictive. This can be a complex problem.

There are organizations, therapists, and books dealing with this subject, and I will not pretend to offer a solution here. Still, even some long-term compulsive snackers have benefited from the following recommendations, all of which are part of the "snacking system" I suggest for *everyone*.

Eat More Vegetables as Snacks

I believe that most people, given a choice between low-nutrient, dense, high-calorie, fatty snacks and tasty nutritious snacks will actually choose the more nutritious ones, *unless* they take more time to prepare. And that is precisely the problem when it comes to eating vegetables as snacks: availability and accessibility. Have you ever noticed how vegetable trays at parties, for example, are always eaten down to the last broccoli stalk? Don't you gobble them down yourself? Most people do, but at home it's a different story. There you are more likely to eat something you can get access to quickly—a few crackers or a yogurt perhaps. A carrot might appeal to you but you don't think about it until it's too late. It would need to be cleaned and prepped. The secret is to take a little time, when you're in the mood, and clean and prepare a supply of fresh vegetables—enough to last a couple of days at a time—or even longer. Properly wrapped, most vegetables will remain crisp for days. Suddenly, with a lot of crunchy vegetables ready to eat, you'll find it easy to pass up those fatty chips and crackers.

Environment over Willpower

Many of my clients complain that they lack the willpower to leave certain snack foods alone, particularly chips and cookies. I tell them that's normal. Environment is stronger than willpower. So *create* the environment that supports your goal. *Replace* the bad snacks with good snacks. Clean out your cupboards and refrigerator, getting rid of the foods you have no control over, whether they are chips, cookies, crackers, or ice cream. Snacks like these are too easy to eat too much of, for *anyone*. And they are so convenient and tempting when we *are* busy and hungry, or in some cases anxious and not hungry, that naturally, we indulge in them—and overindulge—*when they are on hand*. Just see to it that they aren't on hand. Don't buy them, at least not regularly.

Avoid Overeating Healthy Snacks

Many health-conscious snackers oversnack on "good foods," such as cereals, crackers, whole-grain breads, or frozen yogurt. That may be an improvement over chips and cookies, but excessive calories still get stored as fat, even if they are otherwise healthy calories. Figure out how many calories you burn per day by using the chart in Chapter 7. Then keep track of the foods you eat and add up the day's calories. Go ahead and subtract exercise calories. The results may help you control snacking a bit more. It's like figuring out your bank balance to check up on your spending habits. I always make a few less long-distance calls when I review a big telephone bill.

Exercise as Prevention

Exercise can change attitude. For many, it encourages a healthier eating style. When you exercise you feel like eating well. When you eat well you feel like exercising. Why foul up a good thing by stuffing yourself with too many calories after a great workout?

Making It Happen

Make it a goal to eat healthier snacks in the appropriate amounts, and don't forget to include vegetables. Having the right snacks all set to go will make it easier to resist the wrong ones. Then use this system to make it happen:

1. Put your choice of snacks on your shopping list.

2. Go shopping at least once a week and buy most of your food for the week, including fresh vegetables.

3. Prepare the vegetables and fruit either before you put them away, or when you are making a salad at dinnertime. That is a good time to prepare a few extra vegetables for the next day or two.

You may say it takes too much time to shop for an entire week, but it actually takes less time than frequent trips to the store. Once you have all the right food on hand, you won't want to go out to get that Big Mac. *Remember, environment is stronger than willpower.*

SITUATIONAL SNACKING

Snacks at Work or School

I always carry snacks with me. A piece of fruit or a bagel or a box of raisins and a bottle of water, and I'm set. I wouldn't forget them any more than I would forget my purse. In fact, the snack usually gets tossed into my briefcase. Even if I don't end up eating it, it's there. This is good preventive medicine. Vending machines, on the other hand, can be deadly. Choices are improving but are still generally limited to chips, cookies, and candy bars, with an occasional bag of peanuts. Fortunately, fruit is becoming available in some machines. The price you pay for chips, pretzels, nuts, and cheese curls is a snack high in fat, salt, and calories. Choose these snacks only occasionally—once or twice a month.

Snacks at Meetings or Parties

Limit fatty foods at social situations. Decide *ahead of time*—no fat or only moderate fat. Enjoy the experience without depending on huge quantities of food to make the event pleasant. Find someone interesting to talk to; be an interesting person to talk to. Position yourself away from the food in a meeting or cocktail party situation if you can.

When you are the host, take advantage of it. A client of mine named Linda, who has had to struggle with her weight problem, is the office manager for an insurance brokerage company. She meets regularly with insurance agents who use her company as their insurance carrier. Her upcoming schedule included hosting a breakfast meeting for a group of insurance agents. She was planning to serve doughnuts and coffee, because that is what she had always served. It was easy and she thought the others expected it. She would simply make up her mind not to eat any of the doughnuts.

I pointed out to Linda that she was setting herself up: "Poor me, they can eat it, and I can't." Most likely, she would give in. Why not serve one of the breakfasts that got a "10" rating, such as whole wheat bagels, low-fat cream cheese, and apple butter (which is really only a fruit spread with no butter at all)? Linda agreed and decided she would also pick up an assortment of bananas, apples, and oranges, as well as cartons of nonfat fruited yogurt, none of which required any preparation.

Linda later reported the results to me, obviously thrilled. Not only did she feel good about eating half a bagel and an orange, but the insurance agents raved about how much more they liked this breakfast than the old standard breakfast of sweet rolls and coffee. Linda was able to stay true to her new eating style and please those around her. Times are changing.

Snacks at Sporting Events and Movies

These situations set us up for snacking. My client, Peter, is a long-time baseball fan and has season tickets to the San Diego Padres games. This means he goes three or four nights a week when the team is at home. Peter is an accountant with a busy firm. He does everything he can to finish on time on game days, so he can be there for the opening pitch. Arriving hungry and all wound up from a tense day, Peter drinks a beer, eats a hot dog, then popcorn and ice cream every time he goes to a game.

Peter asks me, "Is this okay?" In view of the fact that Peter has put on twenty-five pounds over the past two years, that he is thirty-six with a wonderful family and future ahead of him, and that his father died of heart disease at a young age, the answer is no. Peter is heading in the wrong direction, fast.

I advised Peter, as I have many other clients, to eat *before* going to the game or movie. If that isn't possible, then pick up a sandwich and fruit from a deli on the way to the game. You might have to conceal these items to get through the door or the gate—but that's usually not difficult. Another good choice at the game is a hot pretzel or popcorn without butter if possible.

The No-Dinner Dinner

Appetizers can do more than whet the appetite. They may be appropriately called a light meal in themselves. If you choose to replace dinner with happy hour or snacks, that's okay as long as you make good choices. Stock up on vegetables, go easy on high-fat dips, and choose plain crackers and breads. Forget anything that won't pass the grease test. That means that you can set it on a napkin without a spreading ring of grease around it. Refer to Chapter 15, "Party Snacks" for healthy alternatives to fatty appetizers. Goldfish crackers, popcorn, and pretzels are usually best when eaten in moderate amounts.

Late-Night Snacking

Among the worst nutritional nightmares is out-of-control, late-night snacking. It happens as a reaction to a stressful day, or simply from boredom. The problem late-night snacking produces is threefold: too many calories, poor sleep, and a tendency to skip breakfast. So the cycle is easily repeated the next day. The solution is to eat three meals a day and *stop snacking within an hour or two of bedtime.* Getting back in the breakfast habit is particularly important and particularly effective in curbing those late-night cravings. It may take a few weeks to quell them, but it's well worth the effort.

You'll find most snacks rated at the end of this chapter. For others, see Chapter 8.

DESSERT

I once saw a T-shirt that read, FRUIT IS NOT DESSERT. And I had to agree, at least in part. There are *times* when fruit *is* a satisfying dessert for me, especially during raspberry season or when my neighbor's peach tree is ready, or when cantaloupe with lime and yogurt is served. Often a nice crisp apple or juicy orange is a perfectly satisfying dessert. And again, the theme of environment over willpower applies. If the fruit is being served, great, but if there's also chocolate cake, the competition begins to get steep.

One reason may be the sweet tooth we are born with—in fact it's a key to our survival: an infant becomes oriented to sucking when it seeks out sweetness in breast milk. But there are a myriad of other reasons for our love for rich desserts. The combination of sugar and fat is very satisfying. Perhaps the forbidden pleasure of dessert satisfies our need for self-indulgence. Dessert can even become a reward or a substitute for time off when we're busy, or it may seem to satisfy a need to be taken care of. In fact, studies show that opiate (calming chemical) levels in the brain go up after an infusion of sugar. So we may reach for sweets when we are stressed or pained or lonely.

Although there is nothing wrong with an occasional indulgent dessert, too much fat, sugar, and calories can create new problems.

Fats

The most common fats in desserts are butter, lard, and oils such as palm and coconut. These are the least-desirable fats because they are highly saturated. Cholesterol content of baked goods varies with the type of fat and amount of egg yolk used. Beware of labels that boast cholesterol-free, but contain the saturated vegetable fats that raise cholesterol in the blood. Check labels. Some manufacturers, including Pepperidge Farm, have reformulated their recipes of certain crackers and cookies to replace palm and coconut oils with less saturated oils.

Part of the fat in chocolate is stearic acid, a saturated fat that does *not* appear to raise blood cholesterol. However, the cocoa butter in chocolate is a *saturated* fat. More studies are needed before we are certain how chocolate affects our cholesterol levels. We know, however, that chocolate desserts may be higher in calories, so beware of that aspect. A 1.5-ounce Kit Kat candy bar contains 210 calories, with 11 grams, or 2 teaspoons of fat. The candy bars seem to be getting bigger. If you choose to eat them, look for the smallest ones.

If you bake a chocolate dessert that calls for unsweetened chocolate, substitute three tablespoons of cocoa plus one tablespoon of vegetable oil (such as Puritan) for each one ounce square of chocolate. This cuts down on the saturated fat.

Sugar

Although sugar is not linked to diseases the way fat is, nutritionists recommend limiting it because it provides calories without nutrients. And many high-sugar foods are also high in fat, although in the dessert list at the end of this chapter you will find a few that aren't, like sorbet, popsicles, and fruit ice.

Sweet as it is, sugar has a negative connotation. My seven-year-old niece recently asked me why I—a dietitian—had sugar in my cupboard. I told her about the concept of moderation, that it was okay to eat sugar in small amounts, as long as you ate all the good stuff your body needed. That is true. The problem is, the typical American, including my niece who loves sugar, consumes twenty to thirty teaspoons of sugar a day in different foods and some of that replaces more nutritious foods in her diet. Cutting sugar intake in half is a reasonable goal. Eat more fresh fruits, drink water instead of soda pop or fruit juice, and you'll already be well on your way.

Many dessert labels list other sweeteners that may not sound like sugar but are exactly the same as far as your body is concerned. These include honey, molasses, brown sugar, sucrose, fructose, dextrose, and corn syrup. If several different sugars are listed altogether, sugar may be the item's main ingredient.

Some Desserts that Have Gone on a Diet

Fortunately, our demand for healthy desserts has sparked the introduction of many new alternatives. While it's true that some desserts are never going to be truly "good for you" (even if they are called banana or carrot cake), some new products help us take a bite in the right direction. There are Sara Lee Lights—Double Chocolate Cake and five other frozen varieties with 200 or fewer calories per serving. Pepperidge Farm offers seven varieties in its new frozen dessert line—each had no more than 190 calories and less cholesterol and fat than regular desserts. Hostess cupcakes are now available in a low-fat, no-cholesterol version. The center is filled with jam rather than the creamy filling and thus goes to 7 percent fat from 24 percent.

Many brands of frozen yogurt are touted as healthful stand-ins for ice cream. Their calorie count and fat content, however, vary tremendously and may be higher than ice cream's. Look for those that are available in nonfat and low-fat varieties, and be aware that less fat probably means more sugar—check the calories and, most of all, the portion size. Remember, the toppings of chocolate and nuts add calories, too.

Entenmann's light line of cakes and cookies includes twelve *no-fat* baked products, ranging from Bavarian cream cake to oatmeal raisin cookies. These products use egg whites instead of whole eggs and nonfat milk instead of whole milk as well as different proportions of some other ingredients—generally more sugar. As a result, a two-cookie serving has no fat, instead of the typical 4 grams (36 calories' worth). The pound cake has gone from 115 calories per serving to 80, or as the label boasts "less than 100 calories."

Pay special attention to the serving size in *all* low-calorie products. The dessert may be on a diet, but you won't be if you eat too much of it.

These are occasional options for a fat-free sweet fix, but they are not a dietary "freebie" to be eaten whenever the mood may strike. Plan to include these in your diet when you are not starving.

Moderation, not elimination, is the key. Make your decision. My rating of your favorite dessert may be low, but you may rationalize that you have eaten 8s, 9s and 10s all day, and you can afford a 2. But if you take that rationalization as permission to eat whatever dessert you want *whenever* you want, it is likely to catch up with you.

I suggest that you limit desserts. If you eat them after every lunch and dinner, cut back to once a day. If you eat them once a day, cut back to every other day. Think about what other foods you have eaten in the same day. If you want to fit in more desserts, try to limit your portion size of meat, skip the butter and cheese, and choose desserts, preferably low-fat, only when you have eaten lightly.

To help you make up your mind, ask yourself these questions:

 1. How much have I already eaten today? Can I afford the calories and/or the fat grams?

2. How much did I exercise today? Can I afford the calories?

3. Do I really want this dessert? Is it worth the calories I am spending?

4. When was the last time I ate dessert? Set a goal.

5. If there is an opportunity to select dessert from a tray or a menu, which one is the best choice from a nutritional point of view, while still meeting my need for a treat?

6. Do I really need *this much* dessert? Take the dessert you would normally eat and give half to someone else. Some people say that is only a trigger for a binge, but I find that if I just get a little bit and enjoy it with my tea or coffee, it is all I need to satisfy me. Many of my clients say the same thing.

Here is a list of a few desserts and their ratings. The rich ones average about 70 calories per bite—but if you keep going, the calories add up. For a complete list of dessert ratings, see the chart at the end of this chapter.

	Portion	Rating	Calories
Entenmann's Fat-Free Cookies	3 cookies	6	120
Dreyer's Frozen Yogurt	6 oz.	8	160
Angel food cake	1/9 cake	6	189
Apple pie	1/8	3	282
Vanilla ice cream	3/4 cup	3	550
Giant hot fudge sundae (3 cups ice cream with 1/2 cup syrup and nuts)		3	1342
Cheesecake	3 oz.	2	257

BEVERAGES

Beverages—beer, soda, juices—have become fast foods for many. Just as for solid foods, there are good choices and not-so-good choices. Here's an overview, with ratings at the end of this chapter.

Water

Water is an extremely important nutrient unto itself. Next to air, water is the substance most necessary for survival. Digestion and metabolism of food takes place in a water medium. We can go without food for two or three months, but we can survive only a few days without water. After exercise, a bout with vomiting or diarrhea, or after a salty meal, the simplest, best way to hydrate is with water. Try to drink six to eight glasses a day. (Did you know that as a symptom of dehydration, exhaustion comes before thirst?) Keep a bottle of water in the refrigerator so that you can reach for it instead of a soft drink. Always have water near you when you work. Add a slice of lemon or orange, Bottled waters may have better taste than tap water. Try some.

Soda Pop, Juice Sparklers, and Fruit Punch

These are essentially flavored, sugared water, to the tune of eight to ten teaspoons of sugar and from 120 to 160 calories per twelve-ounce bottle. Even if they are fortified with vitamins A, C, or the latest, calcium, they are not worth the sugar dose. Use them sparingly or not at all.

Noncaloric Sodas and Carbonated Waters

It's not uncommon to see someone wash down a piece of cake with a diet soda or a cup of coffee with artificial sweetener. If the limited use of these products helps to cut down on the amount of sugar you eat, go ahead and use them. But don't use them as an excuse to binge on sugary desserts such as cake or cookies.

Alcohol

Like sugar, alcohol adds calories without adding nutrients. Some evidence links alcohol consumption to development of high blood pressure, which is interesting, because many people claim that alcohol "relaxes" them. In the past few years, many people feel that they have been given the green light to drink an ounce or two of alcohol per day, because studies, however limited, indicated that moderate alcohol increases the HDL cholesterol in the blood, the "good cholesterol." But more recent studies, including a large British one published in *The Lancet* in December 1988, found no positive effect of moderate drinking. In addition, researchers now point out that there are several types of HDL and that the one raised by moderate alcohol intake probably isn't heart-protective.

It is impossible to give specific advice on how much one can safely drink. Most recommendations range from one or two drinks on any given day but no more than six or seven drinks per week. If you have a weight problem, remember that alcohol is a concentrated source of calories, with two beers providing 300 calories, a Scotch and soda 200 calories, and two glasses of white wine around 130 calories, to cite a few examples.

Coffee and Tea

The two concerns here are caffeine, which leads to jittery "coffee nerves," and tannic acids, which may result in stomach problems. Individual reactions to both these substances vary so widely that the best advice is to eliminate these beverages if you have these problems. Fortunately, there is little or no evidence that moderate amounts of coffee affect cholesterol levels. If you choose to drink tea or coffee, limit the strength of the beverage, and keep it to one or two cups per day, preferably before noon.

	Calories	Protein	Fat	Added Sugar	Calcium	Vitamin C
Skim Milk, 8 oz.*	90	8	0	0	200	0
Orange juice, 8 oz.	112	0	0	0	0	97
Low-fat milk, 8 oz	120	8	5	0	297	0
Apple juice, 8 oz.	116	0	0	0	16	2
Diet Coke, 12 oz.	0	0	0	0	0	0
Coke, 12 oz.	155	0	0	8	0	0

*Beverages are not analyzed for caffeine or alcohol content.

CRACKERS, CHIPS, ETC.*

	Rating	Calories	Fat (g)	Saturated Fat (g)	Cholesterol (mg)	Sodium (mg)	Fiber (g)
4 whole-grain rye wafers	8	90	0.4	<.4	<10	230	>1.5
½ large square RyKrisp	8	80	0.4	<.4	<10	224	2.5
3 Pogens Krisprolls	8	120	1.5	<1	<10	<400	>1.5
¾ c. Chex Party Mix, sweet & nutty flavor	8	130	4.1	<2	<10	240	>1.5
½ large square Seasoned RyKrisp	8	100	2.2	<1	<10	294	2.4
4 triple crackers Sesame RyKrisp	8	120	2.8	<1	<4	296	2.1
3 c. Orville Redenbacher's microwave *Light* popping corn, butter/natural flavor	7	60	**2**	<1	0	180	>1.5
2 Chico San rice cakes	7	70	0.4	<.4	<10	0–20	**0.8**
4 Nabisco zwieback crackers	7	120	2	<1	<4	40	<1.5
1 oz. pretzels	7	111	1	<1	<10	451	<1.5
3 c. plain popcorn	7	69	0.9	0	0	0	>1.5
4 pieces Honey Maid Cinnamon or Raisin grahams	7	120	2	<1	0	180	<1.5
4 Nabisco graham crackers	7	120	2	<1	0	180	<1.5
4 squares generic graham crackers	7	120	3	<2	<10	132	<1.5
5 Hain Flavored Mini rice cakes	7	50–60	<1	<.5	0	10–75	<1.5
5 slices New York Style Bagel Chips (original recipe)	7	135	3	<2	0	138	<1.5
5 slices New York Style Bagel Chips (different flavors)	7	135	3	<2	0	288	<1.5
10 saltines	7	130	3	<2	<10	400	<1.5
4 zwieback crackers	7	120	2.4	0.8	<10	72	<1.5

CRACKERS, CHIPS, ETC.* (continued)

	Rating	Calories	Fat (g)	Saturated Fat (g)	Cholesterol (mg)	Sodium (mg)	Fiber (g)
10 soda crackers	7	125	3.7	0.9	<10	312	<1.5
35 oyster crackers	7	116	3.5	0.7	<10	291	<1.5
⅔ c. Chex Party Mix, nacho flavor	7	120	4.3	<3	<10	430	>1.5
⅔ c. Chex Party Mix, regular flavor	7	130	4.7	<3	<10	320	>1.5
3 c. General Mills Pop Secret *Light* microwave popcorn, butter flavor	7	90	4	<1	0	160	>1.5
3 c. Pillsbury Microwave Sugar-coated popcorn†	7	402	3.6	1.2	<10	0	>1.5
6 Nabisco Wheat 'n' Bran Triscuits	6	120	4	<3	0	150	4
6 Nabisco Triscuits	5	120	4	<3	0	150, LS = 70	<1.5
10 Premium saltines	5	120	4	<3	<10	360	<1.5
0.9 oz. Doritos Light tortilla chips, 16 chips	5	110	4	<2	0	250	<1.5
3 c. General Mills Pop Secret microwave popcorn, natural/butter flavor	5	173	10	2	0	323	>1.5
10 Premium Unsalted Tops crackers	5	120	4	<2	<10	230	<1.5
10 Wheatsworth Stone Ground Wheat crackers	5	140	6	<4	<10	270	>1.5
1 oz. Cape Cod Potato Chips, 17 chips	5	150	8	2	<10	150	<1.5
0.9 oz. Doritos tortilla chips, 16 chips	4	140	7	<2	0	250	<1.5
1 oz. potato sticks	4	148	9.8	2.5	0	71	<1.5
3 c. Orville Redenbacher's microwave popping corn, butter/natural flavor	4	100	6	<5	0	290	>1.5
1 oz. Gourmet Microwaveable popcorn	4	106	9	<2	0	0	<1.5
8 Nabisco Waverly crackers	4	140	6	<4	0	320	<1.5
3 c. Pillsbury Microwave Popcorn, salt-free	4	139	5.9	<4	<10	5	<1.5
16 Nabisco Wheat Thins crackers	4	140	6	<4	0	240, LS = 120	<1.5
4 cheese with peanut butter sandwiches	4	139	6.8	1.8	<10	281	<1.5
1 oz. corn chips, 30 small chips, 16 large	4	153	8.8	<6	<10	218	<1.5
1 oz. potato chips, 17 chips	4	148	10.1	2.6	0	133	<1.5
3 c. popcorn with butter & salt	4	123	6	2.7	<10	525	>1.5
10 cheese crackers	3	162	9.8	<8	<50	180	<1.5
1 oz. Pringle's Light Style potato chips	3	147	8.2	<6	0	152	<1.5
14 Nabisco Nutty Wheat Thins	3	140	8	<4	0	340	<1.5
5 pieces cheese straws	3	136	9	3.2	<50	217	<1.5
1 oz. Pringle's Sour Cream 'n Onion potato chips	3	167	13	<10	0	146	<1.5
1 oz. Pringle's regular flavor potato chips	3	167	13	<10	0	215	<1.5
1 oz Pringle's Cheez-ums potato chips	3	167	13	<10	2	240	<1.5

* ALL ENTRIES LOSE ADDITIONAL POINTS FOR LOW VITAMIN AND MINERAL CONTENT.

† LOSES AN ADDITIONAL POINT FOR HIGH SUGAR CONTENT.

NOTE: BOLDFACE NUMBERS INDICATE NUTRITIONAL FACTOR THAT DETRACTS FROM FOOD'S NUTRITIONAL VALUE. (see the note on page 22).

DAIRY SNACKS

DAIRY SNACKS	Rating	Calories	Fat (g)	Saturated Fat (g)	Cholesterol (mg)	Sodium (mg)	Calcium (% U.S. RDA)	Fiber (g)
8 oz. plain skim yogurt w/nonfat dry milk	9	127	0.4	0.3	4	174	45	<1.5
6 oz. Yoplait Light nonfat yogurt w/Nutrasweet	9	90	<1	0	5–7	110	25	<1.5
8 oz. Weight Watchers nonfat fruit yogurt	8	150	<1	0	4	120	25	<1.5
6 oz. Yoplait 150 nonfat yogurt (flavored)	8	150	1	0	5	5	>20	<1.5
6 oz. Light n' Lively low-fat yogurt, fruit flavored	8	170–200	2	—	<10	90–100	20	<1.5
8 oz. low-fat yogurt w/nonfat dry milk, coffee, & vanilla flavors	8	194	2.8	1.8	11	149	39	<1.5
8 oz. plain low-fat yogurt w/nonfat dry milk	8	144	3.5	**2.3**	14	159	42	<1.5
6 oz. Yoplait Low-fat Breakfast Yogurt, 9 flavors	8	228	3.7	—	—	91	—	<1.5
8 oz. low-fat yogurt w/nonfat dry milk, fruit flavored	7	225	2.6	1.7	10	121	**31**	<1.5
1 c. 1% low-fat cottage cheese	6	164	2.3	1.5	10	**918**	14	<1.5
1 c. 2% low-fat cottage cheese	6	203	4.4	**2.8**	19	**918**	16	<1.5
1 oz. hard parmesan cheese	5	111	**7.3**	**4.7**	19	454	34	0
1 oz. Light n' Lively Swiss cheese	4	70	3	**2**	15	350	**20**	<1.5
1 oz. Light n' Lively sharp cheddar cheese	4	70	4	**2**	15	380	**20**	<1.5
1 oz. part skim mozzarella cheese	4	72	**4.5**	**2.9**	16	132	**18**	<1.5
1 oz. Kraft Light Naturals reduced fat cheese	4	84	**5**	**3**	18–21	45–210	25–35	<1.5
¼ c. part skim ricotta cheese	4	86	**5**	**3**	20	78	**16**	<1.5
1 oz. American processed cheese	4	106	**8.9**	**5.6**	27	406	12	0
1 oz. cheddar cheese	4	114	**9.4**	**6**	30	176	**20**	0
1 oz. Monterey cheese	4	106	**8.6**	**>4**	<40	152	**21**	0
1 oz. mozzarella cheese	4	80	**6.1**	**3.7**	22	106	15	0
¼ c. whole milk ricotta cheese	4	108	**8**	**5.2**	32	52	**14**	0
1 oz. Swiss cheese	4	107	**7.8**	**5**	26	74	**27**	0
1 oz. Velveeta Pasteurized Process cheese spread	4	80	**6**	**4**	20	430	15	<1.5
1 oz. Philadelphia Brand cream cheese	3	100	**10**	**5**	30	85	**2**	<1.5
1 oz. Philadelphia Brand lite cream cheese	3	60	**5**	**3**	15	160	**4**	<1.5
1 oz. feta cheese	3	75	**6.0**	**4.2**	25	316	**14**	0
1 oz. Brie cheese	3	95	**7.9**	**>4**	28	178	**5**	0

NOTE: BOLDFACE NUMBERS INDICATE NUTRITIONAL FACTOR THAT DETRACTS FROM FOOD'S NUTRITIONAL VALUE (see the note on page 22).

DESSERTS*

	Rating	Calories	Fat (g)	Saturated Fat (g)	Cholesterol (mg)	Sodium (mg)	Fiber (g)
4 oz. American Glacé, soft serve (all flavors)	8	48	0	0	0	<35	**<1.5**
6 oz. Dreyer's Frozen Yogurt Inspirations (fruit flavored)	8	160	2	—	10	80	**<1.5**
4 oz. Simple Pleasures frozen dessert (all flavors)	7	120–140	<1	<1	5–15	55–90	**<1.5**
¾ c. Dole sorbet, fruit flavors	7	165–180	0.2	0	<15	14–18	**<1.5**
6 oz. Colombo Lite nonfat yogurt	7	143	0	0	0	70	**<1.5**
5 oz. The Country's Best Yogurt (TCBY)	7	150–169	3–4	—	11–15	65	**<1.5**
¾ c. Land o' Lakes fruit-flavored sherbet	7	381	5	3	12	72	**<1.5**
1 Dole fruit & cream bar, varies with flavor	7	90	19	—	5	20	**<1.5**
⅙ Duncan Hines Deluxe carrot cake, from mix	7	374	8	—	0	506	**<1.5**
2 oz. Entenmann's Fat Free Cake (Blueberry Crunch, Chocolate Loaf Cake, Golden Loaf Cake)	7	140	0	0	0	170–260	**<1.5**
2 oz. Entenmann's Fat Free Cake (Lemon Twist Pastry, Banana Crunch, & Pineapple Cheese Coffee Cake)	7	160–190	0	0	0	170–180	**<1.5**
4 oz. Borden/Meadow Gold fat-free frozen dessert (all flavors)	6	90–100	<1	<1	0	40–50	**<1.5**
1 piece homemade angel food cake	6	161	0.1	—	—	161	**<1.5**
⅑ angel food cake, from mix	6	189	0.4	—	—	404	**<1.5**
⅙ Duncan Hines angel food cake, from mix	6	262	0.4	—	0	238	**<1.5**
¾ c. orange sherbet	6	203	3	1.8	11	66	**<1.5**
½ c. Sugar-free Royal pudding, from instant mix	6	103	2.3	—	—	473	**<1.5**
¾ c. vanilla soft-serve ice milk	6	167	4	**2**	10	122	**<1.5**
¾ c. vanilla ice milk	6	138	4.2	**2.6**	14	79	**<1.5**
1 Weight Watchers strawberry cheesecake	6	180	5	1	20	230	**<1.5**
⅙ Duncan Hines Deluxe chocolate chip cake, from mix	6	378	8.8	—	0	498	**<1.5**
3 oz. chocolate fudge	6	339	10.5	**3.6**	—	162	**<1.5**
2 Weight Watchers chocolate brownie	6	200	**6**	2	10	300	**<1.5**
1 Weight Watchers Boston cream pie	6	190	4	1	5	280	**<1.5**
4.5 oz. Honey Hill Farms frozen yogurt	5	118	3.5	—	—	—	**<1.5**
½ c. Royal pudding, from mix	5	162	3.7	—	—	160	**<1.5**
½ c. Royal pudding, from instant mix	5	181	4.4	—	—	375	**<1.5**
6 oz. Yoplait soft frozen yogurt	5	180–200	**6–8**	—	—	50–55	**<1.5**
1 Weight Watchers raspberry mousse	5	150	**6**	<1	5	150	**<1.5**
⅙ Duncan Hines Deluxe devil's food cake, from mix	5	378	8.2	—	0	**726**	**<1.5**
1 Weight Watchers German chocolate cake	5	200	**7**	—	5	190	**<1.5**
⅙ frozen Banquet pumpkin pie	5	197	**8**	—	—	341	**<1.5**
1 Weight Watchers chocolate mousse	5	170	**6**	2	5	190	**<1.5**
1 Jell-O Pudding Pops, vanilla	4	71	2	**1.9**	1	46	**<1.5**
⅙ frozen apple pie	4	231	**9**	2.3	—	195	**<1.5**
1/12 devil's food cake, from mix	4	312	**11.3**	4.4	—	241	**<1.5**
⅛ homemade pumpkin pie	4	241	**12.8**	**4.5**	—	244	**<1.5**
3 oz. chocolate fudge with nuts	4	363	**14.7**	**3.6**	—	144	**<1.5**
⅑ Pillsbury Carrot 'n Spice cake, from mix	4	390	**17**	**—**	—	495	**<1.5**
⅛ Royal cheesecake, from mix	3	225	**9**	**—**	—	370	**<1.5**

DESSERTS* (continued)

	Rating	Calories	Fat (g)	Saturated Fat (g)	Cholesterol (mg)	Sodium (mg)	Fiber (g)
⅛ Royal Lite cheesecake, from mix	3	210	**10**	—	—	380	**<1.5**
1/16 Pillsbury bundt ring, from mix	3	248	**9.8**	—	—	295	**<1.5**
¾ c. regular vanilla ice cream	3	202	**11**	**7**	44	87	**<1.5**
¾ c. Tofu Time Tofutti soft serve	3	237	**12**	—	0	64	**<1.5**
⅛ homemade apple pie	3	282	**12**	—	—	295	**<1.5**
⅛ Jell-O cheesecake, from mix	3	278	**13**	**8**	28	350	**<1.5**
¾ c. rich vanilla ice cream	3	262	**18**	**11**	66	81	**<1.5**
¾ c. Tofu Time Tofutti hard pack (avg. of flavors)	3	330	**20**	—	0	105	**<1.5**
¾ c. vanilla Haagen-Dazs ice cream	3	405	**26**	—	—	220	**<1.5**
Giant hot fudge sundae (3 c. vanilla ice cream, ½ c. chocolate fudge topping, ½ c. whipped cream, ½ oz. chopped walnuts)	3	1342	**77.8**	**42.3**	193	514	**<1.5**
1 Jell-O Pudding Pops, vanilla with chocolate coating	2	127	**7**	**5.5**	1	52	**<1.5**
1 Duncan Hines peanut butter chocolate brownie, from mix	2	150	**8**	—	—	105	**<1.5**
1 Pillsbury microwave fudge brownie	2	190	**9**	—	—	105	**<1.5**
1 Pillsbury microwave fudge brownie with chocolate-flavored chips	2	180	**9**	—	—	110	**<1.5**
⅛ Jell-O banana cream pie, from mix	2	233	**12**	**7.3**	28	267	**<1.5**
¾ c. French vanilla soft-serve ice cream	2	283	**17**	**10**	115	115	**<1.5**
1 piece generic cheesecake	2	257	**16.3**	—	—	189	**<1.5**

* ALL ENTRIES LOSE ADDITIONAL POINTS FOR LOW VITAMIN AND MINERAL CONTENT, AND FOR HIGH SUGAR CONTENT UNLESS LISTED AS SUGAR FREE.
NOTE: BOLDFACE NUMBERS INDICATE NUTRITIONAL FACTOR THAT DETRACTS FROM FOOD'S NUTRITIONAL VALUE (see the note on page 22).

COOKIES*†

	Rating	Calories	Fat (g)	Saturated Fat (g)	Cholesterol (mg)	Sodium (mg)	Fiber (g)
3 Entenmann's Fat-Free oatmeal raisin cookies 3	6	120	0	0	0	125	**<1.5**
3 generic fig bars	6	159	3	—	—	135	**0.2**
3 Nabisco Fig Newtons	6	180	3	—	0	180	**<1.5**
6 generic gingersnaps	6	168	3.6	0.9	—	240	**<1.5**
6 Nabisco gingersnaps	6	180	4.5	—	0	270	**<1.5**
15 generic animal crackers	6	185	3.6	0.9	—	119	**<1.5**
4 generic ladyfingers	6	158	3.4	**1**	—	30	**<1.5**
1 generic molasses	6	137	3.4	0.9	—	125	**<1.5**
3 generic oatmeal raisin	5	176	**6**	**1**	—	63	**<1.5**
6 homemade (recipes vary) sugar cookies	5	213	**8**	**2.1**	—	153	**<1.5**
10 vanilla wafers	4	184	**6.4**	—	—	100	**<1.5**
4 sugar wafers	4	184	**7.4**	**1.8**	—	72	**<1.5**
6 sugar wafers with peanut butter filling	4	198	**8.1**	0.9	—	72	**<1.5**
6 Featherweight wafers (chocolate creme, strawberry creme, & vanilla creme)	4	120	**6**	—	0	0	**<1.5**

COOKIES*† (continued)

	Rating	Calories	Fat (g)	Saturated Fat (g)	Cholesterol (mg)	Sodium (mg)	Fiber (g)
6 Featherweight peanut butter creme wafers	4	150	**6**	—	0	0	**<1.5**
4 Featherweight peanut butter cookies	4	160	**8**	—	0	40	**<1.5**
4 Featherweight cookies (chocolate chip, oatmeal raisin, double chocolate chip, lemon, & vanilla)	4	180	**8**	—	<10	0	**<1.5**
4 Estee assorted creme-filled wafers	4	120	**8**	—	0	20	**<1.5**
3 Estee snack wafers (chocolate, vanilla & strawberry)	3	240	**12**	—	0	15	**<1.5**
2 Estee chocolate-coated snack wafers	3	240	**14**	—	<10	20	**<1.5**
10 generic butter cookies	3	229	**8.5**	—	—	209	**<1.5**
3 generic peanut butter sandwich cookies	3	174	**7**	—	—	63	**<1.5**
3 Pillsbury refrigerated dough sugar cookies	3	201	**8.1**	—	—	192	**<1.5**
3 homemade (recipes vary) oatmeal cookies	3	186	**7.8**	—	—	135	**<1.5**
5 Nabisco Oreos	3	225	**10**	**<5**	—	375	**<1.5**
3 Nabisco Oreos DoubleStuf cookies	3	210	**12**	**3**	—	225	**<1.5**
4 Duncan Hines golden sugar cookies, from mix	3	236	**10**	—	0	132	**<1.5**
3 Duncan Hines oatmeal raisin cookies, from mix	3	201	**9.3**	—	0	95	**<1.5**
4 generic chocolate/vanilla sandwich cookies	3	198	**9**	**2.4**	—	193	**<1.5**
6 generic shortbread cookies	3	225	**10.5**	**1.8**	—	27	**<1.5**
2 generic macaroons	3	181	**8.8**	—	—	225	**<1.5**
4 generic chocolate sandwich cookies	3	196	**8.4**	—	—	252	**<1.5**
3 chocolate-coated graham crackers	3	186	**9.3**	**2.7**	—	159	**<1.5**
4 peanut butter cookies from refrigerated dough	3	200	**10.4**	—	—	228	**<1.5**
3 Duncan Hines peanut butter cookies, from mix	3	203	**11**	—	0	167	**<1.5**
5 Nabisco Party grahams	2	225	**10**	**5**	0	175	**<1.5**
6 Keebler E.L. Fudge cookies	2	210	**9**	—	—	120	**<1.5**
3 Keebler E.L. Fudge sandwich cookies	2	210	**9**	—	—	120–180	**<1.5**
4 generic chocolate chip cookies	2	198	**8.8**	—	—	168	**<1.5**
3 Nabisco Chips Ahoy	2	150	**6**	—	—	120	**<1.5**
5 Pepperidge Farm cookies (Bordeaux, Cappuccino, Chessmen, Milano, Mint Milano, & Orleans)	2	184–217	**8–12**	—	—	58–117	**<1.5**
3 Duncan Hines Double Chocolate cookies, from mix	2	203	**9.3**	—	0	116	**<1.5**
2 Pepperidge Farm cookies (Champagne, Original Pirouettes, Chocolate Laced Pirouettes, Seville, & Paris)	2	200–220	**10–12**	—	—	80–120	**<1.5**
5 homemade shortbread cookies	2	210	**11.5**	—	—	180	**<1.5**
3 Pepperidge Farm cookies (Brussels, Brussels Mint, Geneva, & Orange Milano)	2	170–230	**9–13**	—	—	75–120	**<1.5**
4 homemade (recipes vary) chocolate chip cookies	2	184	**10.8**	—	—	84	**<1.5**
3 Pepperidge Farm cookies (Southport, Capri, Lido, Nassau, & Tahiti)	2	255–270	**13–16**	—	—	75–143	**<1.5**

* ALL ENTRIES LOSE ADDITIONAL POINTS FOR HIGH SUGAR AND LOW VITAMIN AND MINERAL CONTENT.

† PORTION SIZES BASED ON APPROXIMATELY 1.5 OZ. PORTION.

NOTE: BOLDFACE NUMBERS INDICATE NUTRITIONAL FACTOR THAT DETRACTS FROM FOOD'S NUTRITIONAL VALUE (see the note on page 22).

FROZEN DESSERT BARS

	Rating	Calories	Fat (g)	Saturated Fat (g)	Cholesterol (mg)	Sodium (mg)	Fiber (g)
1 Crystal Light bar (diet frozen drink bar)*	7	14	0	0	0	10	**<1.5**
1 Dole Fresh Lites*	7	25	<1	<.5	0	12–30	**<1.5**
1 Dole Fruit 'n Yogurt bar*	7	70	<1	<.5	<5	16	**<1.5**
1 Dole Sun Tops (real fruit juice bar)*	7	40	<1	<.5	0	5	**<1.5**
1 Fruit-A-Freeze Coconut bar*	7	110	1	0	<10	30	**<1.5**
1 Fruit-A-Freeze Pineapple/Strawberry/Watermelon bar*	7	50–90	0–1	0	0	3–25	**<1.5**
1 Weight Watchers sugar-free orange-vanilla treat*	7	30	1	<.5	<5	5	**<1.5**
1 Weight Watchers Chocolate Mint Treat*†	6	60	1	<.5	<5	50	**<1.5**
1 Weight Watchers Chocolate Treat*†	6	100	1	<.5	<5	75	**<1.5**
1 Borden Light Ice Pop*†	6	20	0	0	0	10	**<1.5**
1 Chilly Things Light Pop*†	6	12	0	0	0	5	**<1.5**
1 Knudsen Push-ups (frozen yogurt bars)*†	6	90	1	<.5	<10	25	**<1.5**
1 Weight Watchers vanilla sandwich*†	5	150	3	2	5	170	**<1.5**
1 Creamsicle Sugar Free Cream Pop*	5	25	1	<.5	<5	20	**<1.5**

* LOSES ADDITIONAL POINTS FOR LOW VITAMIN AND MINERAL CONTENT.
† LOSES ADDITIONAL POINT FOR HIGH SUGAR CONTENT.
NOTE: BOLDFACE NUMBERS INDICATE NUTRITIONAL FACTOR THAT DETRACTS FROM FOOD'S NUTRITIONAL VALUE (see the note on page 22).

MILK BEVERAGES

	Rating	Calories	Fat (g)	Saturated Fat (g)	Vitamin A (% U.S. RDA)	Vitamin C (% U.S. RDA)	Calcium (% U.S. RDA)	Sodium (mg)
8 oz. skim milk	9	86	0.4	0.3	10	3	30	126
8 oz. 1% fat low-fat milk	8	102	2.6	**1.6**	10	3	30	123
8 oz. Lactaid low-fat milk	8	102	3	**>1.5**	10	3	30	123
8 oz. chocolate 1% fat low-fat milk	8	158	2.5	1.5	10	3	29	152
10 oz. McDonald's Low-fat Milk Shake (Vanilla, Chocolate, & Strawberry)	8	290–320	1.3–1.7	0.6–0.8	6	<2	35	170–240
10 oz. generic chocolate milk shake	7	356	8.1	**5**	5	0	40	333
8 oz. 2% fat low-fat milk	6	121	**4.7**	**2.9**	10	3	30	122
8 oz. chocolate 2% fat low-fat milk	6	179	5	**3.1**	10	3	29	150
8 oz. hot cocoa prepared w/water	6	103	1.1	0.7	<1	**2**	**10**	149
10 oz. generic vanilla milk shake	6	350	9.5	**5.9**	7	0	46	299
8 oz. 3.5% fat whole milk	5	150	**8**	**4.9**	7	8	29	122
8 oz. chocolate whole milk	4	208	**8.5**	**5.3**	6	3	28	149
1 tbsp. strawberry flavored mix in 8 oz. whole milk	4	234	**8.2**	**5.1**	6	3	29	128
8 oz. hot cocoa prepared w/whole milk	4	218	**9.1**	**5.6**	6	3	30	123
8 oz. nonalcoholic eggnog	3	342	**19**	**11.3**	18	7	33	138

NOTE: BOLDFACE NUMBERS INDICATE NUTRITIONAL FACTOR THAT DETRACTS FROM FOOD'S NUTRITIONAL VALUE.

FRUIT/VEGETABLE JUICES AND JUICE DRINKS

	Rating	Calories	Fat (g)	Saturated Fat (g)	Vitamin A (% U.S. RDA)	Vitamin C (% U.S. RDA)	Calcium (% U.S. RDA)	Sodium (mg)
8 oz. fresh orange juice	9	111	0.5	0.1	10	207	3	2
8 oz. Citrus Hill Plus Calcium orange juice from concentrate	9	120	<1	0	<10	160	27	0
8 oz. fresh pink grapefruit juice	9	96	0.3	0	22	157	2	2
8 oz. canned orange juice	9	104	0.5	0.1	9	143	2	6
8 oz. orange juice from frozen concentrate	9	112	0.4	0.1	4	162	2	2
8 oz. canned grapefruit juice	9	93	0.2	0	<1	120	2	3
8 oz. grapefruit juice from frozen concentrate	9	102	0.3	0	<1	138	2	2
8 oz. canned carrot juice	9	97	0.4	0.2	1260	35	6	72
8 oz. fresh yellow passion fruit juice	9	149	0.4	0.1	119	75	1	15
8 oz. grape juice from frozen concentrate	9	128	0.2	0.1	<1	100	1	5
4 oz. fruit juice with 6 oz. club soda	9	56	0	0	0	50	1	4
8 oz. pineapple juice from frozen concentrate	9	129	0.1	0	1	50	3	3
8 oz. Campbell's V-8 vegetable cocktail, no salt added	9	53	0	0	85	86	41	55
8 oz. canned tomato juice cocktail	9	51	0.2	0	39	65	2	486
8 oz. canned apricot nectar	9	141	0.2	0	66	2	2	9
8 oz. Dole New Breakfast Juice (average of flavors)	9	120	0	0	<10	133	<5	11
8 oz. sugar-free orange Tang from powder	9	7	0	0	13	133	3	2
8 oz. bottled cranberry juice cocktail	8	147	0.1	0	<10	180	1	10
8 oz. Campbell's V-8 vegetable cocktail	8	49	0.1	0	67	82	3	**789**
8 oz. canned vegetable juice cocktail	8	45	0.3	0	57	111	3	**883**
8 oz. canned tomato juice	8	43	0.1	0	27	73	2	**875**
8 oz. canned peach nectar	8	134	0.1	0	13	22	1	17
8 oz. canned papaya nectar	8	142	0.4	0.1	6	13	2	14
8 oz. orange Tang from powder	8	117	0	0	13	133	8	4
8 oz. apple juice from frozen concentrate	7	111	0.3	0	<1	2	1	17
8 oz. canned/bottled apple juice	7	116	0.3	0	<1	3	2	7
8 oz. canned/bottled grape juice	7	155	0.2	0.1	<1	0	2	7
8 oz. sugar-free Country Time lemonade	7	5	0	0	0	15	3	0
8 oz. Crystal Light lemonade, from powder	7	5	0	0	0	10	<5	0
8 oz. sugar-free Kool-Aid, from powder	7	3	0	0	0	12	<10	8
8 oz. Country Time lemonade, from powder	6	82	0	0	0	15	<5	21
8 oz. Kool-Aid, from powder	6	98	0	0	0	10	<10	8

NOTE: BOLDFACE NUMBERS INDICATE NUTRITIONAL FACTOR THAT DETRACTS FROM FOOD'S NUTRITIONAL VALUE (see the note on page 22).

SODAS & MISCELLANEOUS BEVERAGES	Rating	Calories	Fat (g)	Saturated Fat (g)	Vitamin A (% U.S. RDA)	Vitamin C (% U.S. RDA)	Calcium (% U.S. RDA)	Sodium (mg)
12 oz. club soda	7	0	0	0	<2	<2	2	75
12 oz. diet cola	7	1	0	0	<2	<2	<2	1–20
12 oz. Tab cola	7	1	0	0	<2	<2	<2	8
12 oz. Diet Sprite	7	4	0	0	<2	<2	<2	0
12 oz. Diet Slice	7	26	0	0	<2	<2	<2	11
12 oz. brewed black tea	7	4	0	0	<2	<2	<2	10
12 oz. brewed coffee	7	8	0	0	<2	<2	<2	8
12 oz. tonic water/quinine water	6	125	0	0	<2	<2	<2	15
12 oz. ginger ale	6	124	0	0	<2	<2	<2	25
12 oz. lemon-lime soda	6	149	0	0	<2	<2	<2	41
12 oz. regular cola	6	151	0	0	<2	<2	<2	14
12 oz. root beer	6	152	0	0	<2	<2	<2	49
12 oz. cherry cola	6	164	0	0	<2	<2	<2	5
12 oz. orange soda	6	177	0	0	<2	<2	<2	46
12 oz. Mountain Dew	6	179	0	0	<2	<2	<2	31
12 oz. General Foods International Coffee, sugar-free, from instant powder (Amaretto, Cappuccino, Francais, Irish Creme, Irish Mocha Mint, Orange Cappuccino, Suisse Mocha, & Vienna)	5	54–72	**3.8–5.2**	**3.4–4.2**	<2	<2	<2	36–190
12 oz. General Foods International Coffee, sugar sweetened, from instant powder (same flavors as above)	4	102–124	**3.8–5.2**	**3.4–5.2**	<2	<2	<2	38–212

NOTE: BOLDFACE NUMBERS INDICATE NUTRITIONAL FACTOR THAT DETRACTS FROM FOOD'S NUTRITIONAL VALUE (see the note on page 22).

CHAPTER · 7

THE FAST-FOOD WEIGHT-LOSS PLAN

FAST-FOOD, SENSIBLE WEIGHT LOSS

A weight-loss plan using fast foods? Absolutely. I've set out to bridge the gap between the ideal weight-loss diet and the demands of our busy lives. And I've succeeded. My many clients will attest to that. My fast-food plan produces *sensible, gradual, lasting* weight loss.

The first attempt many people make at weight loss is to "stop eating" one or more meals altogether—usually breakfast or lunch. Then they eat enough at dinner to put them right back into calorie overload. When these "home" methods fail, the dieter begins shopping for a more structured diet program. When people come to me, they are often at wits' end with all the programs they have tried. Perhaps they have been on a diet program of severely restricted food intake combined with "support" meetings. Or they have been having daily sessions with a counselor (usually one without formal training in nutrition) who weighs them and parcels out their food for the day. Many have tried liquid diets to avoid dealing with food and eating altogether, often losing weight and gaining it back. Almost all have been baffled and frustrated by their doctors simplistic advice: "Eat less and exercise more."

The client confesses a sense of hopelessness, and blames himself/herself for lack of "willpower."

To understand your overeating, you must understand yourself. Sometimes, psychotherapy may be appropriate. But over the years, I've seen far too many people erroneously label themselves "food addicts," the victims of an eating disorder, when the real problem is the way they manage their lifestyles. In fact, they let their lifestyle manage them. They need help changing eating habits in a satisfying way *within* those lifestyles.

It's a fact that a particularly busy lifestyle can promote weight gain. "No time to exercise." "No time to eat right." Those are the complaints I hear over and over again. This book has already demonstrated that it is possible—in fact, easy—to "eat right" in a hurry. It's also possible—again, easy—to get enough exercise, and to do so in an enjoyable way, even with the busiest schedule. More on that soon. First let's tackle the food issue.

When we live fast and eat food on the run, it's very easy to eat too much, especially too much fat. In addition, we are commonly served huge portions with twice as much food as we need. Just ask the Japanese who move here, discover the American diet of burgers, fries, fried fish and chicken, and bacon and eggs. They soon develop the same problems we have—overweight and diseases of overconsumption. Although McDonald's has outlets all over Japan, the high-fat diet has not become a way of life for Japanese yet. They indulge in "American food" as an occasional meal, while maintaining their traditional diet: steamed rice, vegetables, and fish, with steak as a luxury, all in smaller portions than would ever be served in an American restaurant. We would do well to turn the table, and adapt their diet as a mainstay, and ours as the occasional treat!

So what is the answer? Fortunately, as we've already seen, it's getting easier all the time to eat in a healthy fashion—fast. Many restaurants offer more variety of salads and entrées prepared with less fat, even promoted as "light" or "heart-healthy" alternatives. Fast-food restaurants are responding to our requests for healthier, lighter fare with salads, salad bars, and chicken sandwiches which are often grilled instead of breaded and deep-fried. Many restaurants serve low-fat milk as their standard. A continental breakfast on the airplane used to consist of sweet rolls and coffee. The new continental breakfast may be a choice of cereal and fruit, or yogurt and a bagel. You can even register your fruit-bagel request with your frequent-flier plan. What we lack in motivation, as discussed in the preceding chapter, we are finally beginning to make up for by creating a low-fat, low-calorie environment.

THE FAST-FOOD MENU PLANS

The Fast-Food Diet weight-loss plan is concerned not only with calories, but also with the *balance* of calories from carbohydrate, protein, and fat, as well as healthy amounts of fiber, cholesterol, and sodium. This chapter provides you with daily meal plans with top ratings (7, 8, 9, 10) that can be eaten at home or ordered in a restaurant. It is best not to switch meals (lunch and dinner, for example), but you can switch days around. This will ensure a balance of nutrients. You can repeat the menus until you make progress with your weight goals and feel comfortable with the new style of eating, or you can use your own menus. How much weight you lose will depend on your metabolic rate and your exercise level.

The common denominator of most unsuccessful diets is that they have tried to restrict your calories *too much*. You must be realistic about your need for food. I see many men, tall men in particular, who sabotage their weight-loss efforts by adapting the 800- or 1,000-calorie levels of their female dieting partners. This is too low a calorie level for a man. Even if a man could stay with it, he is likely to lose as much lean body mass (muscle) and water as fat. In addition, his metabolic rate could decrease by as much as 20 percent. Then, when he returns to his usual calorie intake, he will *gain* weight at the same calorie level that he formerly maintained his weight.

We all want results fast. But fast weight loss is neither healthy nor is it likely to be maintained. If you have had these experiences in the past, learn from them. Don't set yourself up for failure by putting yourself on a short-term deprivation program.

To choose your appropriate calorie level, you must estimate your body's energy or calorie needs. Very generally speaking, your calorie need will depend on your sex, your height, and your activity level. Four different calorie-level selections are provided: 1,000, 1,250, 1,500, and 1,800 calories. For women who are less than five feet five inches, 1,000 to 1,250 calories is generally appropriate. I suggest 1,250 to 1,500 calories for women over this height, depending on calorie expenditure from exercise. For men who are five feet seven inches or less, the 1,250- to 1,500-calorie plan is recommended. Men over this height should eat no less than 1,500 to 1,800 calories, depending on size and their exercise routine. A typical exercise workout that burns 300 calories per session five times a week will help achieve a reasonable fat weight loss—a half pound of fat per week.

If an extremely heavy exercise routine is undertaken (one that burns 1,500 to 2,000 calories, as in running a twenty-six-mile marathon, or cycling one hundred miles), more food must be eaten or lean muscle will be burned for fuel. My twenty-two-year-old client, Kevin, played rugby for San Diego State University. At a height of six feet four inches, weighing 236 pounds, and having 23 percent body fat, he came to me with the goal of building muscle and losing fat. After careful record keeping, calorie counting, and body-composition testing, we determined that Kevin required 2,600 calories per day without exercise and 4,860 calories per day with his workout program (three to five hours each day). If Kevin had restricted his intake to

1,800 calories, he would never have been able to reach his goal of gaining muscle. In fact, he would have lost muscle along with the fat. By eating 3,700 to 3,800 calories per day, he was taking in 1,000 less than he was burning. With his trainer's well-planned aerobic and weight-lifting routine, Kevin was able to lose 29 pounds of fat and gain 5 pounds of lean muscle in six months, for new figures of 212 pounds at 12 percent body fat. He looks great, and feels great out on the rugby field.

A fairly accurate way to determine calorie expenditure is to keep records of food and exercise and monitor weight and body-composition changes. This can be tedious, but it's well worth the time and effort if you have difficulty losing weight. You will need to buy a book of the calorie content of foods in order to do this. Another way to count calories is by using the exchange lists from the American Diabetes Association. These lists categorize foods into groups with assigned calorie values to specific portions of foods. (A registered dietitian can help you do this—check the Yellow Pages for one nearest you, and be sure you work with someone who has "R.D." after his or her name.)

Some people have lower metabolic rates and may have a difficult time losing weight. This may be because they do not exercise enough or because they have been restricting calories for a long time, or a combination of both. This pattern of restrained eating puts the body into a state of starvation, and the body reacts by slowing down its metabolic rate in order to conserve fat stores. Sad, but true, it is often these dieters who have been most faithful to low-calorie plans who find themselves in this difficult position—that of needing so few calories that they must eat less food than another person (of the same size) while still only maintaining their weight or perhaps even continuing to gain weight. In my clinical experience, I see this as a problem particularly in small women, five feet, four inches or less.

If you fall into this category, it is especially important for you to avoid very low-calorie diets and to rely more on exercise for weight loss (which will be slow). Exercise can also help to increase your lean body mass, and consequently, increase your metabolic rate. Avoid the very low-calorie diets, whether they are liquid or from regular food, because they will only compound your problem and add to the risk of further lowering your metabolic rate.

Although I suggest that you choose from four calorie levels, ranging from 1,000 to 1,800, it is best to consult an expert—registered dietitian or your doctor—before you begin, particularly if your metabolism is atypical or your level of exercise burns more than 300 to 500 calories per day.

The Fast-Food Diet offers a *variety* of foods, important for a diet for life. By including a vast array of foods you love to eat, in the appropriate amounts, you can enjoy eating and never tire of your menu choice. The goal is to eat healthfully because you *prefer* it that way.

The composition of the diet is as follows:

 50 to 60 percent carbohydrate (emphasizing complex carbohydrate and fiber)

20 to 30 percent fat (with 7 percent polyunsaturated and 7 percent monounsaturated, 7 percent saturated fat)

15 to 20 percent protein

300 milligrams of cholesterol or less

2,400 milligrams of sodium

20 to 30 grams of fiber

These guidelines are similar to those recommended by the American Heart Association, the American Cancer Institute, National Cholesterol Education Program, and National Research Council.

Asterisks at the end of entries refer to recipes that can be found in the book.

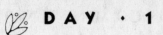

	CALORIE LEVEL			
BREAKFAST	1,000	1,250	1,500	1,800
Nutri-Grain cereal	½ cup	1 cup	1 cup	1 cup
Whole wheat toast	1 slice	1 slice	2 slices	2 slices
Jam	1 tsp.	1 tsp.	2 tsp.	2 tsp.
Low-fat milk[1]	½ cup	½ cup	1 cup	1 cup
LUNCH				
Tuna Salad on Whole Wheat[1]*				
Tuna salad[2]	2 oz.	2 oz.	3 oz.	3 oz.
Banana	1	1	1	1
Snack: apple	1	1	1	1
Water or noncaloric beverage				
DINNER				
Barbecued Chicken Breasts with Tabasco and Lime*	3 oz.	3 oz.	3 oz.	4 oz.
Rice	½ cup	½ cup	1 cup	1½ cups
Whole wheat roll	1	1	1	1
Light margarine	1 tsp.	1 tsp.	2 tsp.	2 tsp.
Broccoli	½ cup	1 cup	1 cup	1½ cups
Snack: popcorn	3 cups	3 cups	3 cups	6 cups
Water or noncaloric beverage				

FAST-FOOD NOTES: 1. We chose low-fat milk because many people prefer it on their cereal, but if you have already made the switch to nonfat milk, stay with it. 2. At lunch, your tuna salad sandwich prepared according to the recipe in Chapter 11 will have one-third less the calories of the traditional tuna salad sandwich because we have added extra vegetables and used light mayonnaise.

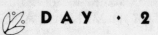 **D A Y · 2**

	CALORIE LEVEL			
BREAKFAST	1,000	1,250	1,500	1,800
Bagel[1]	½	1	1	1
Light margarine or cream cheese	1 tsp.	2 tsp.	2 tsp.	2 tsp.
Orange	1	1	1	1
Low-fat milk	—	—	1 cup	1 cup
LUNCH				
Chicken sandwich[2]				
Last night's chicken	2 oz.	3 oz.	3 oz.	3 oz.
Whole wheat bread	2 slices	2 slices	2 slices	2 slices
Light mayonnaise	2 tsp.	1 tbsp.	1 tbsp.	1 tbsp.
Lettuce, tomato				
Apple	—	—	—	1
Snack: Quaker Honey and Oat bar	—	1	1	1
Water or noncaloric beverage				
DINNER				
Greens with Red Onion and Citrus	1 cup	1 cup	1 cup	1 cup
Pan-Sautéed Snapper[3] with Mushrooms and Bell Peppers*	3 oz.	3 oz.	3 oz.	4 oz.
Baked potato	½ med.	1 med.	1 med.	1 med.
Green beans	1 cup	1 cup	1 cup	½ cup
Low-fat milk	1 cup	1 cup	1 cup	1 cup
Light margarine	1 tsp.	2 tsp.	1 tbsp.	1 tbsp.
Snack: Quaker Honey and Oat bar	—	—	—	2

FAST-FOOD NOTES: 1. Bagels are a great way to start your day, providing complex carbohydrates without the fat in a croissant or a doughnut. 2. To make your meals most efficient we suggest that you make your lunch out of last night's dinner whenever possible. If it doesn't work out that way, try to select a sandwich that is similar to the one in the menu plan. Commercially available grilled chicken sandwiches are available at Wendy's, McDonald's, Hardee's, Burger King, and Carl's Jr. 3. You will notice we have included fish on your menu at least three times a week to provide you with valuable fish oils.

	CALORIE LEVEL			
BREAKFAST	1,000	1,250	1,500	1,800
Oatmeal[1]*	1 cup	1 cup	1 cup	1 cup
Raisins	1 tbsp.	1 tbsp.	1 tbsp.	1 tbsp.
Low-fat milk	½ cup	1 cup	1 cup	1 cup
LUNCH				
Tortilla stuffer[2]*				
Last night's fish	2 oz.	3 oz.	3 oz.	3 oz.
Corn tortilla	1	2	2	2
Lettuce, cabbage, or tomato				
Low-fat mozzarella cheese	—	—	—	1 oz.
Banana	1	1	1	1
Water or noncaloric beverage				
Snack: frozen fruit bar	1	1	1	1
DINNER				
Basic Tossed Green Salad with Vinaigrette*	1 cup	1 cup	1 cup	1 cup
Barbecued Teriyaki Flank Steak[3]*	3 oz.	3 oz.	4 oz.	4 oz.
Fried Rice with Zucchini and Mushrooms*	½ cup	1 cup	1 cup	1 cup
Water or noncaloric beverage				
Snack: graham crackers	—	2	4	6
Low-fat milk	—	—	½ cup	1 cup

FAST-FOOD NOTES: 1. The fiber in oatmeal may help to lower cholesterol in your blood, so we suggest that you include it once a week at breakfast. The old-fashioned variety is our favorite but the instant oatmeal is fine and can be mixed in a mug at the office. 2. A major objective of the Fast-Food menu plan is to decrease the portion size of your animal protein throughout the day. Consequently, we have a hunch that you will have leftover fish for today's lunch. 3. Beef for dinner? Yes it's true that beef can be included in a low-fat diet when a lean cut of meat is chosen, the cooking method limits added fat, and the portion size is kept at three ounces. This is easy to do with the stir-fry in tonight's dinner.

	CALORIE LEVEL			
BREAKFAST	1,000	1,250	1,500	1,800
Whole wheat toast	1 slice	2 slices	2 slices	2 slices
Peanut butter[1]	2 tsp.	1 tbsp.	1 tbsp.	1 tbsp.
Orange juice	½ cup	1 cup	1 cup	1 cup
Banana	—	—	1	1
LUNCH				
Turkey sandwich[2]				
Turkey	2 oz.	2 oz.	3 oz.	3 oz.
Whole wheat bread	2 slices	2 slices	2 slices	2 slices
Alfalfa sprouts				
Low-fat cheese of choice	—	—	1 oz.	1 oz.
Tomato				
Light mayonnaise	2 tsp.	2 tsp.	1 tbsp.	1 tbsp.
Carrot	1	1	1	2
Water or noncaloric beverage				
DINNER				
Spinach salad or tossed green	1 cup	1 cup	1 cup	2 cup
Light Italian salad dressing	2 tsp.	1 tbsp.	1 tbsp.	1 tbsp.
Spaghetti with Marinara Sauce*				
Pasta Marinara sauce (see option: bottled sauce, or	1 cup	1½ cups	2 cups	2 cups
fresh tomato, both listed on recipe)	⅓ cup	½ cup	¾ cup	¾ cup
Parmesan cheese	2 tsp.	2 tsp.	1 tbsp.	1½ tbsp.
Garlic bread	1 slice	1 slice	1 slice	2 slices
Light margarine	1 tsp.	2 tsp.	2 tsp.	1 tbsp.
Water or noncaloric beverage				
Snack: Graham Crackers	1	1	1	1

FAST-FOOD NOTES: 1. High-fat foods like peanut butter can be handled in three ways: we can eliminate them. We can substitute an alternative version of the same food. Or we can eat less of them. We have chosen to include peanut butter because it is a good source of niacin, magnesium and protein and a favorite of many. Note that the portion size is limited. 2. Turkey sandwiches are probably your safest best when our lunch suggestion is not manageable for you. When the sandwich is prepared according to the amount specified on the menu above, a low-fat sandwich is the perfect combination to keep your energy level high in midafternoon.

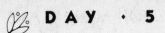

DAY · 5

	CALORIE LEVEL			
BREAKFAST[1]	1,000	1,250	1,500	1,800
Strawberries	1 cup	1 cup	1 cup	1 cup
Nutri-Grain cereal	1 cup	1 cup	1 cup	1 cup
Low-fat milk	½ cup	1 cup	1 cup	1 cup
LUNCH				
Last night's pasta	1 cup	1½ cups	1½ cups	2 cups
Salad greens	1 cup	1 cup	1 cup	1 cup
Light Italian dressing	2 tsp.	2 tsp.	1 tbsp.	1 tbsp.
Water or noncaloric beverage				
Snack: Seasoned RyKrisp crackers	6	6	12	12
Apple	1	1	1	1
DINNER				
Baked Potato Stuffed with Ricotta Cheese[2]*	1 med.	1 med.	1 large	1 large
Light margarine	1 tsp.	1 tsp.	1 tsp.	1 tsp.
Nonfat plain yogurt	1 tbsp.	1 tbsp.	1 tbsp.	1 tbsp.
Steamed carrots and cauliflower with dill	1 cup	1 cup	1 cup	1 cup
Water or noncaloric beverage				
Snack: Dreyer's Light ice cream, Sealtest Free or Knudson Free nonfat frozen dessert[3]	—	½ cup	½ cup	1 cup

FAST-FOOD NOTES: 1. Meeting one's need for fiber is tricky these days, since we are often faced with white rice, sourdough bread, and too few vegetables. Breakfast is a perfect opportunity to get a dose of fiber—a good reason not to skip it, even if it means carrying it with you and eating it midmorning rather than first thing in the day, especially when you have eaten late the night before—not an ideal situation but something that happens in the real world. 2. Low-fat ricotta cheese is the protein source in this meatless dinner. Notice it is followed by a heavier breakfast. You are learning to "think thin"! 3. You will notice that the Fast-Food menus use "light" products such as low-fat or nonfat ice cream, salad dressing, margarine, mayonnaise, and various cheeses. As consumers, we are fortunate to have so many alternatives, along with the assurance (at last!) from the federal government that any food labeled "light" must actually contain one-third fewer calories than their respective counterparts.

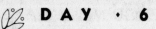

	CALORIE LEVEL			
BREAKFAST	1,000	1,250	1,500	1,800
French Toast[1]*	2 slices	2 slices	2 slices	2 slices
Light syrup	2 tsp.	2 tsp.	2 tsp.	1 tbsp.
Light margarine	2 tsp.	2 tsp.	1 tbsp.	1 tbsp.
Orange juice	½ cup	½ cup	1 cup	1 cup
LUNCH				
Tuna Pocket Sandwich[2]*				
Tuna	2 oz.	3 oz.	3 oz.	4 oz.
Light mayonnaise	2 tsp.	2 tsp.	1 tbsp.	1 tbsp.
Pita	1	1	1	1
Water or noncaloric beverage				
Snack: low-fat cheese	1 oz.	1 oz.	1 oz.	2 oz.
RyKrisp crackers	4	6	8	8
DINNER				
Cajun Chicken*	3 oz.	3 oz.	3 oz.	4 oz.
Zucchini-Carrot Stir-Fry*	1 cup	1 cup	1 cup	1½ cups
Potato Fries[3]*	½ cup	1 cup	1 cup	2 cups
Low-fat milk	1 cup	1 cup	1 cup	1 cup
Snack: apple	1	1	1	1

FAST-FOOD NOTES: 1. French toast is a great weekend breakfast, especially when prepared the Fast-Food way (here without the fruit sauce), resulting in fewer calories, fat, and cholesterol, with more fiber, vitamins and minerals. 2. At lunchtime, experiment with different types of breads—pita is suggested here, choosing whole grains as often as possible. Then continue the good choice theme by limiting the portion size of protein inside your sandwich. 3. The potato fries suggested with the barbecued chicken can be made from leftover baked potatoes, Day 5, just remember to prepare a few extras. Then simply cut them up to look like your favorite french fry, and pan-fry them in a nonstick pan with one teaspoon of diet margarine. Once they are brown, add a sprinkle or two of water to steam them along. Add a sprinkle of parsley for color and serve with traditional catsup.

	CALORIE LEVEL			
BREAKFAST	1,000	1,250	1,500	1,800
Bagel	1	1	1	1
Light cream cheese[1]	2 tsp.	2 tsp.	1 tbsp.	1 tbsp.
Orange juice	½ cup	½ cup	1 cup	1 cup
LUNCH				
Peanut Butter and Jelly Sandwich*				
Whole wheat bread	2 slices	2 slices	2 slices	2 slices
Jelly	2 tsp.	1 tbsp.	1 tbsp.	1 tbsp.
Peanut butter	2 tsp.	1 tbsp.	1 tbsp.	1 tbsp.
Banana	1	1	1	1
Low-fat milk	½ cup	1 cup	1 cup	1 cup
Snack: fig bar	1	1	2	3
DINNER				
Mozzarella and Tomato Pizza[2] with Spinach*	¼	½	½	½
or Weight Watchers Combination Pizza Dinner	½	1	1	1
Garlic bread	2 slices	2 slices	2 slices	2 slices
Margarine	1 tbsp.	1 tbsp.	1 tbsp.	1 tbsp.
Green salad	1 cup	1 cup	1 cup	2 cups
Light dressing	2 tsp.	2 tsp.	1 tbsp.	1 tbsp.
Water or noncaloric beverage				
Snack: Frozen yogurt or Dreyer's Light ice cream	½ cup	½ cup	1 cup	1 cup

FAST-FOOD NOTES: 1. Cream cheese is like peanut butter—it's a high-fat food we can choose to eliminate, eat small amounts of, or as we have chosen here, to substitute a "light" alternative form which has one-third fewer calories. Stay with your good choice by keeping the portion size small. Try putting it on, then scraping it off—so you can actually see the bagel through the cream cheese, just enough to season and moisten your bagel. 2. Pizza can be a perfect food—the crust as a complex carbohydrate, the veggies as vitamins, and a touch of cheese for the protein and familiarity. The key is the amount of cheese. If you order this pizza in a restaurant, try "no cheese" on half the pizza—just for the experience! If you won't go that far, at least ask for light cheese: eight ounces of cheese on medium pizza will cut the calories by one-third.

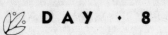

	CALORIE LEVEL			
BREAKFAST	1,000	1,250	1,500	1,800
Shredded wheat	1 cup	1 cup	1 cup	1½ cups
Banana	1	1	1	1
Low-fat milk	½ cup	1 cup	1 cup	1 cup
LUNCH				
Turkey sandwich				
Turkey	2 oz.	2 oz.	3 oz.	3 oz.
Part-skim mozzarella cheese	—	—	1 oz.	1 oz.
Light mayonnaise	2 tsp.	2 tsp.	1 tbsp.	1 tbsp.
Whole wheat bread	2 slices	2 slices	2 slices	2 slices
Lettuce, tomato				
Nectarine	1	1	1	1
Water or noncaloric beverage				
Snack: oatmeal cookie	1	2	2	2
Low-fat milk	—	—	½ cup	1 cup
DINNER				
Baked Swordfish Steaks with Lemon, Tomato and Cracked Peppercorns[1]*	3 oz.	3 oz.	3 oz.	4 oz.
Baked potato	1 med.	1 med.	1 med.	1 large
Asparagus	1 cup	1 cup	1 cup	1 cup
Light margarine	2 tsp.	1 tbsp.	1 tbsp.	1 tbsp.
Water or noncaloric beverage				
Snack: peach	1	1	1	1
Frozen yogurt or Dreyer's Light ice cream, or Sealtest Free or Knudson Free nonfat frozen dessert		½ cup	½ cup	¾ cup

FAST-FOOD NOTES: 1. Many people enjoy fish in restaurants but don't cook it at home. We encourage both: you will enjoy fish at home if you make sure it is fresh, nicely seasoned, and not overcooked. The rule of thumb is the same whether you bake, broil, or poach your fish: ten minutes per inch. Season with a lemon, dill, and our wonderful "cream sauce."

	CALORIE LEVEL			
	1,000	1,250	1,500	1,800
BREAKFAST				
Cinnamon toast	2 slices	2 slices	2 slices	2 slices
Light margarine	2 tsp.	2 tsp.	1 tbsp.	1 tbsp.
Low-fat milk	½ cup	½ cup	1 cup	1 cup
Sliced strawberries	—	1 cup	1 cup	1½ cup
LUNCH				
Chili[1]*	1 cup	1 cup	1 cup	1½ cups
Rye Krisp Crackers, triples	4	4	6	6
or				
Saltines, doubles	4	4	6	6
Snack: Apple	1	1	1	1
Graham crackers	—	4	4	8
DINNER				
Chicken Stir-Fry[2]* (or Chinese take-out—moo goo gai pan w/chicken and vegetable)	1 cup	1½ cup	2 cups	2½ cups
or Chicken Breast	3 oz.	3 oz.	4 oz.	4 oz.
Fried Rice with Zucchini and Mushrooms[3]*	1½ cups	2 cups	2 cups	3½ cups
Low-fat milk	½ cup	1 cup	1 cup	1 cup
Snack: Fortune cookie	1	1	1	1

FAST-FOOD NOTES: 1. Chili can be prepared from the recipe on page 198 or picked up at Wendy's. Our recipe has more beans and therefore more fiber, whereas Wendy's has more meat and fat, but the calories are comparable, and both fit in with recommended goals for total daily fat and calorie intake. 2. The dinner of chicken stir-fry will keep your protein portion in line. 3. Be careful when choosing the vegetables for your dish—as we increase the overall vegetables in your diet, it is possible to become tired of so many. Limiting vegetables to two or three varieties per stir-fry will make you less likely to repeat veggies and will require less preparation time.

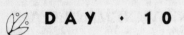

	CALORIE LEVEL			
BREAKFAST	1,000	1,250	1,500	1,800
Nutri-Grain cereal	1 cup	1 cup	1½ cups	1½ cups
Low-fat milk	½ cup	1 cup	1 cup	1 cup
Banana	1	1	1	1
Whole wheat toast	—	—	—	1 slice
Light margarine	—	—	—	2 tsp.
LUNCH				
Tuna sandwich				
Tuna	2 oz.	3 oz.	3 oz.	4 oz.
Whole wheat bread	2 slices	2 slices	2 slices	2 slices
Light mayonnaise	2 tsp.	1 tbsp.	1 tbsp.	1 tbsp.
Lettuce, tomato				
Orange	1	1	1	1
Water or noncaloric beverage				
Snack: frozen yogurt or Dreyer's light ice cream	½ cup	½ cup	1 cup	1 cup
Oatmeal cookie	—	—	1	2
DINNER				
Salad greens	1 cup	1 cup	1 cup	2 cups
Light Italian dressing	2 tsp.	1 tbsp.	1 tbsp.	1 tbsp.
Turkey Burgers[1]*				
Ground turkey	3 oz.	3 oz.	4 oz.	4 oz.
Onion roll	1	1	1	1
Light mayonnaise	2 tsp.	1 tbsp.	1 tbsp.	1 tbsp.
Lettuce, tomato				
Water or noncaloric beverage				
Snack: popcorn	—	2 cups	2 cups	3 cups

FAST-FOOD NOTES: 1. Turkey burgers are a perfect solution to backyard barbecues. Guests love to know that healthy food can taste good, too! These made a big hit at a Super Bowl party I put together. Season your meat with onion, red and green bell peppers, garlic, soy sauce, black pepper, and fresh parsley or cilantro. (See Chapter 14 for exact cooking instructions.) The three-ounce turkey burger provides 2½ teaspoons of fat, whereas a burger made from lean ground beef would provide 3½ teaspoons—a 25 percent savings. Whether you choose beef or turkey, the more major issue becomes cheese and sauce. Hold them!

	CALORIE LEVEL			
BREAKFAST	1,000	1,250	1,500	1,800
Oatmeal	1 cup	1 cup	1 cup	1½ cups
Orange	1	1	1	1
Low-fat milk	½ cup	1 cup	1 cup	1 cup
LUNCH				
Chicken salad sandwich				
Chicken salad	¼ cup	½ cup	½ cup	½ cup
Bagel	1	1	1	1
Apple	1	1	1	1
Water or noncaloric beverage				
Snack: string cheese	—	—	2 oz.	2 oz.
Wheatsworth crackers	—	6	6	8
DINNER				
Lean Cuisine Zucchini Lasagna[1]	1	1	1	1
Basic Tossed Green Salad with Vinaigrette*	½ cup	1 cup	1 cup	1 cup
Whole wheat or onion roll	1	1	1	2
Light margarine	2 tsp.	2 tsp.	2 tsp.	1 tbsp.
Water or noncaloric beverage				
Snack: Dreyer's Light ice cream	—	—	½ cup	1 cup

FAST-FOOD NOTES: 1. Frozen dinners have made a comeback in the past few years, with low-fat, rather tasty entrées that say "no" for the dieter. Portion control is a major objective for the individual trying to lose weight and these dinners help in that regard. We caution against using the frozen dinners too frequently due to their high sodium content, but we include them here to bridge the gap between "ideal" and "practical." The list below, in fact, meets the criteria for a sensible diet: 300 calories or less, no more than 30 percent of calories from fat, 1,000 milligrams or fewer of sodium and 15 grams or more of protein.

Healthy Choice: Sole au Gratin
Benihana Oriental Light: Chicken in Spicy Garlic Sauce
Budget Gourmet, Slim Selects: Oriental Beef and Oriental Vegetables
Le Menu Light Style Dinners: 3-Cheese Stuffed Shells
Stouffer's Lean Cuisine: Zucchini Lasagna
Weight Watchers: Pasta Rigati in Meat Sauce

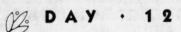 **DAY · 12**

	CALORIE LEVEL			
BREAKFAST	1,000	1,250	1,500	1,800
Honeydew melon	1 cup	1½ cups	1½ cups	2 cups
Whole wheat English muffin	1	1	1	1
Peanut butter	2 tsp.	1 tbsp.	1 tbsp.	1 tbsp.
Low-fat milk	½ cup	1 cup	1 cup	1 cup
LUNCH				
Turkey sandwich				
Turkey	2 oz.	3 oz.	3 oz.	3 oz.
Onion roll	1	1	1	1
Part-skim mozzarella cheese	—	—	1 oz.	1 oz.
Lettuce, tomato				
Light mayonnaise	2 tsp.	1 tbsp.	1 tbsp.	1 tbsp.
Water or noncaloric beverage				
Snack: Carrot & celery sticks	4	4	6	6
Cucumber yogurt dip	1 tbsp.	2 tbsp.	3 tbsp.	4 tbsp.
DINNER				
Fajitas with Chicken (or lean beef) and Bell Peppers[1]*				
Chicken breast	3 oz.	3 oz.	4 oz.	5 oz.
Corn tortillas	1	2	2	3
Green pepper, onion				
Oil for stir-frying	1 tsp.	1 tsp.	2 tsp.	1 tbsp.
Rice	1 cup	1 cup	1½ cups	1½ cups
Water or noncaloric beverage				

FAST-FOOD NOTES: 1. If you choose to order the steak fajitas in your favorite Mexican restaurant, ask for your dinner to be prepared with minimal oil. Take a good look at your food when it arrives and consider the portion size recommended on your plan. Share your dinner with someone, or take half of it home and enjoy the next day—remember restaurants almost always serve at least two times the amount you need.

	CALORIE LEVEL			
BREAKFAST	1,000	1,250	1,500	1,800
Shredded wheat	1 cup	1 cup	1 cup	1 cup
Low-fat milk	1 cup	1 cup	1 cup	1 cup
Banana[1]	½	½	½	1
LUNCH				
Low-fat cheese[2]	1 oz.	2 oz.	2 oz.	3 oz.
RyKrisp crackers	4	6	8	8
Apple slices	2	4	4	4
Raw carrot	1	1	1	1
Water or noncaloric beverage				
Snack: microwave popcorn[3]	—	1 cup	2 cups	2 cups
DINNER				
Chicken Parmesan with Pasta*				
Chicken	3 oz.	3 oz.	3 oz.	3 oz.
Pasta	½ cup	1 cup	1 cup	1½ cups
Green Beans Vinaigrette	½ cup	1 cup	1 cup	1 cup
Water or noncaloric beverage				
Snack: Fruit sherbet or frozen yogurt	—	—	2 cups	2 cups

FAST-FOOD NOTES: 1. The vitamin C in your morning fruit or juice will help you to absorb the iron in your whole grain or occasional egg. Yes, you should be taking a basic vitamin-mineral supplement whenever you are restricting your calories, but it is still important to rely on foods for nutrients most of the time. 2. Although you may not need a recipe for cheese and crackers, we urge you to review our recipe for cheese and crackers found in Chapter 11. You will see how your choice of a low-fat cheese and low-fat cracker can cut the fat and calories in half. 3. Microwave popcorn is all the rage these days, so we took a trip to the supermarket and scrutinized the label on a few of the most popular brands and here is the scoop:

  Orville Redenbacher, butter flavored, 2 cups = 67 calories, 4 grams of fat; light = 40 calories, 1.3 grams of fat
  Jolly Time, 2 cups = 90 calories, 3.6 grams of fat
  Pop Secret, 2 cups = 116 calories, 6.7 grams of fat; light = 60 calories, 2.7 grams of fat

Mr. Redenbacher appears to be the best in choice both in terms of total calories, and percentage of calories from fat, although variations are not drastic. The key here becomes eating two to three cups rather than the entire bag.

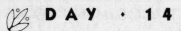

	CALORIE LEVEL			
BREAKFAST	1,000	1,250	1,500	1,800
Oatcakes[1]* (or Nutrigrain frozen waffles)	2	2	2	3
Low-fat milk	½ cup	½ cup	1 cup	1 cup
Light margarine	2 tsp.	1 tbsp.	1 tbsp.	1 tbsp.
Light syrup or	2 tsp.	1 tbsp.	1 tbsp.	2 tbsp.
Applesauce	½ cup	½ cup	½ cup	½ cup
LUNCH				
Last night's chicken	2 oz.	3 oz.	3 oz.	4 oz.
Pasta	½ cup	1 cup	1 cup	1½ cups
Water or noncaloric beverage				
Snack: frozen yogurt	—	½ cup	1 cup	1 cup
DINNER				
Shrimp with Garlic[2]*	4 oz.	4 oz.	5 oz.	6 oz.
Baked potato	1 med.	1 med.	1 med.	1 large
Light margarine	2 tsp.	2 tsp.	1 tbsp.	1 tbsp.
Water or noncaloric beverage				
Nonfat plain yogurt	—	—	2 tsp.	1 tbsp.

FAST-FOOD NOTES: 1. Portion size is a major issue with pancakes. A short stack in a restaurant may easily yield 400 to 600 calories before the butter and syrup are added. Visualize a pancake equal to the size of a small slice of bread—eat the equivalent of one or two, omit the butter, and go easy on the topping. Fruit topping is a great alternative to syrup. Puree a ripe banana, an orange, a squeeze of lemon, and ¼ cup raisins soaked for a few minutes in ½ cup boiling water. It is sure to be a big hit. Make this your style of eating pancakes—while you are losing weight and once you are at your weight goal. 2. Shrimp has a reputation for being a high-cholesterol food. But researchers have done some recalculating in the past few years and have determined that 3 ounces of shrimp contains only about 147 milligrams of cholesterol, compared to 213 milligrams in one egg or about 73 milligrams in 3 ounces of chicken. That's somewhat high but not outrageous. In addition, the shrimp is very low in saturated fat, which is a major factor in raising blood cholesterol. You should know your own blood cholesterol and make a decision about your daily dietary cholesterol quota based on your dietitian's advice.

	CALORIE LEVEL			
BREAKFAST	1,000	1,250	1,500	1,800
Grape-Nuts cereal	¼ cup	½ cup	½ cup	¾ cup
Low-fat milk	½ cup	1 cup	1 cup	1 cup
Banana	½	½	½	1
Whole wheat toast	1 slice	1 slice	1 slice	1 slice
Light margarine	1 tsp.	1 tsp.	1 tsp.	1 tsp.
LUNCH				
Last night's shrimp in tortillas				
Shrimp	3 oz.	4 oz.	6 oz.	6 oz.
Corn tortilla	1	1	2	2
Tomato salsa	¼ cup	¼ cup	¼ cup	¼ cup
Water or noncaloric beverage				
Snack: graham crackers	4	4	4	6
Peanut butter	2 tsp.	2 tsp.	2 tsp.	2 tsp.
Apple	—	1	1	1
DINNER				
Salad greens	1 cup	1 cup	1 cup	2 cups
Lite salad dressing	2 tsp.	2 tsp.	2 tsp.	2 tsp.
Corn Chowder with Potato Soup[1]* (or Progresso				
Vegetable Beef)	1 cup	1 cup	2 cups	2 cups
Dinner roll	1	1	1	2
Light margarine	2 tsp.	2 tsp.	2 tsp.	1 tbsp.
Water or noncaloric beverage				

FAST-FOOD NOTES: 1. Dovetailing is an art involving the use of a leftover food from one day delightfully disguised the next day. Case in point is the leftover baked potato in the corn chowder soup, my favorite! So quick with frozen corn and a food processor. Adjust the amount of milk to the desired consistency, and puree only part of the corn, for an interesting texture.

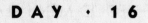

	CALORIE LEVEL			
BREAKFAST	1,000	1,250	1,500	1,800
Mixed fresh fruit[1]	½ cup	1 cup	1 cup	2 cups
Low-fat plain yogurt	¼ cup	½ cup	1 cup	1 cup
Whole wheat toast	1 slice	1 slice	1 slice	2 slices
Light margarine	1 tsp.	1 tsp.	1 tsp.	2 tsp.
Water				
LUNCH				
Peanut Butter and Jelly Sandwich[2]*				
Whole wheat bread	2 slices	2 slices	2 slices	2 slices
Peanut butter	2 tsp.	2 tsp.	2 tsp.	1 tbsp.
Jelly	2 tsp.	1 tbsp.	1 tbsp.	1 tbsp.
Banana	1	1	1	1
Low-fat milk	½ cup	½ cup	1 cup	1 cup
Snack: low-fat cheese	1 oz.	1 oz.	2 oz.	2 oz.
Wheatsworth crackers	6	6	6	6
DINNER				
Chicken w/ 2 tsp. bottled barbecue sauce or recipe (page 209)	3 oz.	3 oz.	4 oz.	4 oz.
Corn-on-the-cob	1	1	1	1
Spinach salad	1 cup	1 cup	1 cup	2 cups
Light margarine	1 tsp.	1 tsp.	1 tsp.	1 tsp.
Light salad dressing	2 tsp.	2 tsp.	1 tbsp.	1 tbsp.
Water or noncaloric beverage				
Snack: Dreyer's Light ice cream, Sealtest Free or Knudson Free nonfat frozen dessert	—	¾ cup	1 cup	1 cup

FAST-FOOD NOTES: 1. Fruit for breakfast is great but contrary to the popular "Fit for Life" diet recommending fruit only until noon, we do need a bit of protein and complex carbohydrates to keep the blood-sugar level stable. For many people, the "Fit for Life" diet was an improvement over their own eating habits, and because the recommendations are basically healthy and result in fewer calories, people may lose weight. But the premise of food combining to change metabolic activity has no scientific basis, and there is no need to give the digestive system a rest during the morning hours. 2. If your lunch meals are eaten at the office, you may want to keep an inventory of a few easy-to-prepare foods—good old-fashioned peanut butter and jelly may save you from a poorer selection in a pinch.

	CALORIE LEVEL			
BREAKFAST	1,000	1,250	1,500	1,800
Nutri-Grain cereal	1 cup	1 cup	1 cup	1 cup
Raisins	1 tbsp.	1 tbsp.	1 tbsp.	1 tbsp.
Low-fat milk	½ cup	1 cup	1 cup	1 cup
Whole wheat bagel	—	—	½	1
Light margarine	—	—	1 tsp.	2 tsp.
LUNCH				
Ham sandwich				
Lean ham[1]	2 oz.	3 oz.	3 oz.	3 oz.
Dinner roll	1	1	1	1
Lettuce, tomato				
Apple	—	—	1	1
Water or noncaloric beverage				
Snack: Kellogg's Rice Krispies bar	—	—	—	1
DINNER				
Fettuccine with Clam Sauce[2]*	1½ cups	2 cups	2 cups	2 cups
Salad greens	1 cup	1 cup	1 cup	1 cup
Light Italian dressing	2 tsp.	2 tsp.	2 tsp.	1 tbsp.
Garlic toast (option: Roman Grilled Garlic Toast with Roma Tomatoes*)	1 slice	1 slice	2 slices	2 slices
Light margarine	2 tsp.	2 tsp.	2 tsp.	1 tbsp.
Water or noncaloric beverage				

FAST-FOOD NOTES: 1. Lean ham can be almost as low in fat as chicken when it is truly lean. Select it as an alternative, limit the ham to two to three ounces, and substitute mustard for mayonnaise. Lettuce, tomato, sprouts, and a cucumber will add a crunch without many calories. Just be sure to skip the cheese, chips, and pickle and avoid high-sodium foods the remainder of the day. 2. A can of chopped clams and a bit of spaghetti is easily turned into a delightful dinner—truly fast food at home, and great again as tomorrow's lunch.

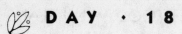

	CALORIE LEVEL			
	1,000	1,250	1,500	1,800
BREAKFAST				
English muffin[1]	1	1	1	1
Jam	2 tsp.	2 tsp.	1 tbsp.	1 tbsp.
Light margarine	1 tsp.	1 tsp.	2 tsp.	2 tsp.
Cantaloupe	—	½	½	¾
LUNCH				
Last night's pasta with clam sauce	1½ cups	2 cups	2 cups	2½ cups
Garlic toast	—	—	2 slices	2 slices
Turkey sandwich (see Day 8)	1	1	1	1
light margarine	—	—	2 tsp.	2 tsp.
Water or noncaloric beverage				
Snack: Nonfat or low-fat fruit yogurt	6 oz.	6 oz.	6 oz.	8 oz.
Fig bar or Rice Krispies bar	—	—	—	2
DINNER				
Salad greens	1 cup	1 cup	1 cup	2 cups
Light salad dressing	2 tsp.	2 tsp.	1 tbsp.	1 tbsp.
Fresh Tomato Pizza*	⅛	⅙	⅙	⅙
or Weight Watchers Pizza	1	1	1	1
Water or noncaloric beverage				

FAST-FOOD NOTES: 1. How are your whole grains holding up? Review your choices the past few days and aim for at least 50 percent of grain choices as whole grains. Whole wheat English muffins are available, and you may find a whole wheat pizza crust on a rare occasion. Just keep in mind the extra vitamin B-6, zinc, and fiber (not to mention flavor) that whole grains provide and you will be motivated to seek them out whenever possible.

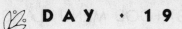 **D A Y · 1 9**   FAST-FOOD MENU PLANS

	CALORIE LEVEL			
BREAKFAST	1,000	1,250	1,500	1,800
Shredded wheat	1 cup	1 cup	1 cup	1 cup
Low-fat milk	1 cup	1 cup	1 cup	1 cup
Banana	1	1	1	1
Bagel	—	½	½	1
Light cream cheese	—	—	2 tsp.	2 tsp.
Jam	—	2 tsp.	2 tsp.	2 tsp.
LUNCH				
Bean Nut Butter Sandwich[1]*	1	1	1	1
Whole wheat pita	1	1	1	1
Water or noncaloric beverage				
Snack: nonfat or low-fat fruit yogurt	6 oz.	6 oz.	6 oz.	8 oz.
Oatmeal cookie[2]	—	—	2	2
DINNER				
Cuban-style Beef in Tortilla*	2 oz.	3 oz.	3 oz.	4 oz.
Corn tortilla	1	2	2	2
Salad greens	1 cup	1 cup	1 cup	1 cup
Light salad dressing	2 tsp.	2 tsp.	1 tbsp.	1 tbsp.
Low-fat milk	—	½ cup	1 cup	1 cup
Snack: microwave popcorn	2 cups	2 cups	2 cups	3 cups

FAST-FOOD NOTES: 1. Now here is an alternative sandwich for you! We have substituted a bean dip for the meat or cheese. Be sure to plan an extra snack in the afternoon particularly if you plan to exercise at the end of the day because this low-fat sandwich may leave you hungry in midafternoon. 2. It is a common belief that one must eliminate all sweets in order to lose weight, but this is simply untrue. Total calorie balance is the issue, and sweets must be included in this perspective (there's that word again!). We chose a cookie as a sweet because it is generally lower in fat and calories than such goodies as cakes, pies, or candy bars—choose the small crunchy variety of cookies, which may provide 100 to 150 calories. If you can't trust yourself with a bag of cookies—don't buy them. Pick up one cookie at the corner store.

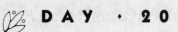

	CALORIE LEVEL			
BREAKFAST	1,000	1,250	1,500	1,800
Oatmeal	1 cup	1 cup	1 cup	1½ cups
Raisins	1 tbsp.	1 tbsp.	1 tbsp.	1 tbsp.
Low-fat milk	1 cup	1 cup	1 cup	1 cup
Whole wheat toast	1 slice	1 slice	2 slices	2 slices
Light margarine	1 tsp.	1 tsp.	1 tsp.	1 tbsp.
Banana	—	—	1	1
LUNCH				
Tuna salad sandwich				
Tuna	3 oz.	3 oz.	4 oz.	6 oz.
Pita	1	1	1	1
Lettuce, tomato				
Light mayonnaise or low-fat yogurt	2 tsp.	1 tbsp.	1 tbsp.	1 tbsp.
Water or noncaloric beverage				
Snack: frozen fruit bar	1	1	1	1
or fig bar	—	—	—	2
DINNER				
Zucchini with Onions, Tomatoes, and Basil[1]*	2 cups	3 cups	3 cups	3 cups
Garlic toast	1 slice	2 slices	2 slices	2 slices
Light margarine	1 tsp.	2 tsp.	1 tbsp.	1 tbsp.
Salad greens	1 cup	1 cup	1 cup	2 cups
Light Italian salad dressing	2 tsp.	2 tsp.	2 tsp.	1 tbsp.
Water or noncaloric beverage				
Snack: Low-fat cheese	—	2 oz.	2 oz.	2 oz.
Crackers	—	4	4	6

FAST-FOOD NOTES: 1. Now that you are getting adjusted to less animal protein, we would like to challenge you with a dinner with no animal protein. Remember, everything that grows contains a certain amount of protein. Since most Americans eat two to three times the protein they need, there is rarely a concern of too little protein. Here, a slice of part-skim mozzarella cheese will provide animal protein—note it is an "added touch" rather than the main focus of the meal.

	CALORIE LEVEL			
BREAKFAST	1,000	1,250	1,500	1,800
Scrambled Eggs with Spinach in a Pita[1]*	1	2	2	2
Whole wheat pita or tortilla	2	2	2	2
Orange juice	½ cup	1 cup	1 cup	1 cup
LUNCH				
Last night's zucchini	1 cup	1 cup	1 cup	1½ cups
Pita	1	1	1	1
Part-skim Mozzarella cheese	1 oz.	1 oz.	1 oz.	1 oz.
Water or noncaloric beverage				
Snack: grapes	½ cup	½ cup	1 cup	1½ cups
DINNER				
Roasted turkey breast	3 oz.	3 oz.	3 oz.	4 oz.
Mashed sweet potatoes	½ cup	½ cup	1 cup	2 cups
Light margarine	2 tsp.	2 tsp.	1 tbsp.	1 tbsp.
Water or noncaloric beverage				
Snack: Wheatsworth crackers	2	2	6	8
Peanut butter	2 tsp.	2 tsp.	1 tbsp.	1 tbsp.
Low-fat milk	—	—	—	1 cup

FAST-FOOD NOTES: 1. Eggs at last—if you like them. This recipe cuts the cholesterol in half by using only one yolk with two whites. (1 yolk = 213 mg. cholesterol) The spinach adds a nice touch of flavor and nutrition, wrapped in a whole-grain pita or tortilla, this is a delightful weekend breakfast that your family or friends will enjoy. Your calcium intake is important, which is why we have included one to three servings of dairy products on each day's menu. The Recommended Dietary Allowance for calcium is in the process of being increased from 800 milligrams to 1,200 milligrams. Consider that one cup of milk contains about 300 milligrams of calcium and add a calcium carbonate or gluconate supplement to meet your needs. Also, remember that exercise and hormones play an equally important role in the irreversible process of bone loss.

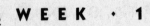

WEEK · 1   SHOPPING LIST

Remember to check your items already on hand against the shopping list!

DAY	ITEM	DAY	ITEM
PRODUCE, FRUITS, & VEGETABLES		**CANNED & BOTTLED GOODS**	
1, 2, 3, 7	Salad greens	1, 7	Jams
1	Tomato	1	Water-packed tuna
1, 4	Banana	1, 2	Light mayonnaise
1	Lime	1	Tabasco sauce
1, 5, 6	Apple	2	Rice vinegar
1	Garlic	4, 7	Peanut butter
1, 3	Broccoli	4	Light Italian salad dressing
2	Orange		Bottled Ragu spaghetti sauce
2	Red onion	6	Cajun seasoning
2, 3	Bell peppers		Olive oil
2	Potatoes, red		Puritan oil
2, 6	Green beans		
3	Banana	**BAKERY & DELI ITEMS**	
3	Ginger	1, 2, 4	Whole wheat bread
2, 3, 4	Mushrooms	1	Whole wheat roll
4	Alfalfa sprouts	2, 7	Bagel
4, 5	Carrot	3	Corn tortilla
4	Spinach	4	Sliced turkey
4	Zucchini		
5	Strawberries	**FROZEN FOODS**	
5, 6	Baking potato	2, 4, 6	Orange juice
		3	Frozen Fruit bar
CEREALS, GRAINS, PASTAS, BEANS		3	Pineapple juice concentrate
1, 5	Nutri-Grain cereal	5, 7	Dreyer's Light ice cream
1	Rice	7	Weight Watchers Combination Pizza
	Wine for cooking	7	Frozen yogurt
1	Nutri-Grain bar		
2, 7	Fig bars	**DAIRY & EGGS**	
3	Oatmeal	3, 5, 6, 7	Low-fat milk
3	Raisins		Light margarine
3	Graham crackers	4	Parmesan cheese
4	Spaghetti	4	Nonfat or low-fat fruit yogurt
5	Seasoned RyKrisp	2, 6, 7	Light cream cheese
		3	Part-skim mozzarella cheese
FISH, POULTRY, & MEAT			
1, 2, 6	Chicken		
2	Snapper		
3	Flank steak		

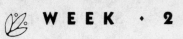
Remember to check your items already on hand against the shopping list!

DAY	ITEM	DAY	ITEM

PRODUCE, FRUITS, & VEGETABLES

DAY	ITEM
8, 10, 13	Banana
8	Nectarine
8, 14	Baking potato
8	Asparagus
8	Tomato
8, 11	Lemon
8	Peach
9	Zucchini
9, 11, 13	Apple
10, 11	Orange
10, 11	Salad greens
12	Cucumber
12	Lime
12	Garlic
12	Honeydew melon
12, 13	Carrot
12	Celery
12	Green bell pepper
12	Onion
13	Green beans

CEREALS, GRAINS, PASTAS, BEANS

DAY	ITEM
8	Shredded wheat
8, 10	Oatmeal cookie
9, 12	Rice
10	Nutri-Grain cereal
10, 13	Popcorn
11, 14	Oatmeal
11, 13	Wheatworth crackers
13	Pasta
13	Quaker Honey and Oat bar

FISH, POULTRY, & MEAT

DAY	ITEM
8	Swordfish or other white fish
9, 13	Chicken breast
10	Ground turkey
12	Flank steak
14, 15	Shrimp

CANNED & BOTTLED GOODS

DAY	ITEM
8	Olive oil
9	Salsa
9	Wine vinegar, red and white
10	Water-packed tuna
11	Chicken
12	Peanut butter
14	Light syrup

BAKERY & DELI ITEMS

DAY	ITEM
8, 12	Sliced turkey
8, 9, 10	Whole wheat bread
9, 12	Corn tortilla
10	Onion roll or hamburger bun
11	Bagel
12	Whole wheat English muffin

FROZEN FOODS

DAY	ITEM
10	Light ice cream
11	Lean Cuisine Zucchini Lasagna
13	Fruit sherbet
8, 10, 13, 14	Frozen yogurt

DAIRY & EGGS

DAY	ITEM
8, 11, 13	Low-fat milk
	Part-skim mozzarella cheese
12	Nonfat plain yogurt
14	Eggs

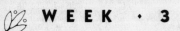

Remember to check your items already on hand against the shopping list!

DAY	ITEM
PRODUCE, FRUITS, & VEGETABLES	
15, 16, 19	Banana
15, 17, 18	Salad greens
15	Potato
16	Corn on cob
16, 18, 21	Spinach greens
17	Peach
18	Cantaloupe
18, 20	Garlic
18	Pizza veggies
	Mushrooms
18, 20	Peppers
18, 20	Basil
18, 20	Spinach
18, 20	Onion
20	Tomato
20	Zucchini
21	Grapes
21	Sweet potatoes
CEREALS, GRAINS, PASTAS, BEANS	
15	Grape-Nuts cereal
15	Graham crackers
16	Wheatworth crackers
17	Nutri-Grain cereal
	Raisins
17	Kellogg's Rice Krispies bar
17	Fettuccine
19	Shredded wheat
19	Oatmeal cookie
FISH, POULTRY, & MEAT	
16	Chicken
19	Lean ground beef
	Turkey

DAY	ITEM
CANNED & BOTTLED GOODS	
15	Salsa
	Peanut butter
	Jam
16	Barbecue sauce
17	Clams
18	Pizza sauce
19	Garbanzo beans
20	Water-packed tuna
20	Olive oil
	Dijon mustard
	Basil or oregano
	28-ounce can whole tomatoes
BAKERY & DELI ITEMS	
15, 19	Corn tortilla
15, 17	Dinner roll
15, 16, 20	Whole wheat bread
17	Sliced ham
18	Sliced turkey
18	Whole wheat English muffin
20, 21	Whole wheat pita bread
FROZEN FOODS	
18	Weight Watchers Pizza
15	Corn
20	Frozen fruit bar
16	Dreyer's Light ice cream
DAIRY & EGGS	
16, 18, 20	Plain low-fat yogurt
17	Mozzarella cheese
17	Parmesan cheese
18, 19	Nonfat or low-fat fruit yogurt
	Pillsbury pizza crust
21	Eggs

TIPS ON MAKING PERMANENT CHANGES

The following lifestyle changes will support you in losing weight now and in managing your weight forever.

Limit access to certain foods: Get rid of those foods in your snacks that are eaten with a fork or a spoon. How about baked goods, cheese, or nuts? If they are problem foods for you, you don't need them in your house. Ask for support from other family members to help you through the initial stages of change.

Plan meals in advance and make sure they are satisfying: People who binge may be in a stronger position if they consider meals that are balanced, as opposed to replacing meals with a single food such as popcorn or vegetables or cereal.* Create meals with adequate cupboards that are likely to sabotage your diet. If it's finger foods like cookies, chips, and crackers, dump them. Instead, plan meals and amounts of complex carbohydrates, which promote meal satiety, *and* fat, which slows the time it takes for food to leave the stomach, enhancing the feeling of fullness. A balance of food also increases satiety, so include vegetables, salads, fruit, and whole-grain breads. The fiber in foods helps to increase the sensation of fullness, and often increases the time it takes to eat your meal. Warm foods tend to be more satisfying than cold foods or foods eaten at room temperature.

Stop eating when you are full: Eating an appropriate amount is important. Check my portion sizes listed on the Fast-Food Diet menu plans. If you are a poor judge, then get out your measuring cup and measure your cereal before you put it in the bowl. You won't need to do it more than once or twice if you use the same bowl. Weigh your chicken, fish, or other animal protein on a scale to check its size. Then, when you are in a restaurant, you can estimate by sight. If you don't already have a food scale, invest in one. They are available at many supermarkets as well as at gourmet food stores.

If eating the right amount is extremely difficult for you, you will get extra help from foods that are naturally divided into portions, such as potatoes (rather than rice or pasta), six- to eight-ounce containers of yogurt or ice cream, precut meats, and frozen dinners and entrées.

Pay attention to your stomach. Before you reach for another piece of bread, think about it. Do you really need it? Don't be a slave to your habits. Put yourself in control. Have you had enough to eat? If so, *stop* eating.

Relax for a few minutes before eating: This helps put you in the best frame of mind to really enjoy your food and eat less. Or,

---

* C.L. Rock and J. Yager, "Nutrition and Eating Disorders: A primer for clinicians," *International Journal of Eating Disorders* 6 (1987): 276.

exercise before eating to relieve the day's stress. It may not always be possible to set aside the time, but do it when you can. Resolve to eat meals and snacks sitting down. Then, whether it's a short pause and a deep breath, or reading the newspaper, figure out what will help you reach a relaxed state before you begin eating. Use food appropriately: to meet your nutritional needs rather than to reduce your stress level.

When you finish eating in a restaurant, ask the waiter or waitress to take your plate away. If you are at home, by yourself, push yourself away from the table and go for a walk around the block. Should you find yourself overeating, try to think about what happened and do some problem solving. Ask yourself these questions: "What did I want this food to do for me?" "Did I want it to relieve boredom, fatigue, stress, pressure?" "What nonfood activity would have been a better way to manage my mood?"

It's true that we all find ourselves under stress from time to time. It's difficult, if not impossible, to eliminate stress completely, so the key is to change the way we *react* to stressful situations. Managing stress by overeating is only likely to create a new stress.

It is interesting to note how different people react differently to food. The anorexia patient gives me the same reason for undereating as the overweight patient gives me for overeating. My client, Lisa, has battled anorexia nervosa for the past five years. She complains that she loses weight when she goes on a vacation because she is distracted and forgets to eat. This is the opposite of Kathy's problem. She puts on weight during her vacation because she lets her guard down and eats too many calories.

Clearly, it is not the situation alone that makes us eat more or less, it is how we have learned to react to the situation. And since it is learned, it can be *unlearned* or modified, and replaced with a new, more positive response. But it takes awareness and persistent effort.

You must also allow yourself to be human. Your ideal may not come all at once. People who try to give up cigarettes, for example, generally have two to three relapses before they succeed, usually occurring within the first three months. The same is even more likely to happen with food, since unlike the cigarette habit, we do have to eat! But lapses and relapses simply mean that it's time to start over again. Try to learn something from these experiences. Was the fattening food really a treat?

If food has become very important to you, to the extent that you are constantly thinking about it, you must find other pleasurable activities. Sure, you may continue to enjoy food and find it a source of comfort and enjoyment. But try to supplement your life with nonfood activities. Get involved in a project in your home, volunteer to feed the hungry, go for a walk, or read a book.

Keep a record of food and exercise: My clients who commit to the tedious task of record keeping tend to do much better than those who can't be bothered. Use it as a tool to review the past and set goals for future eating behaviors. The form that follows should help you.

DAILY FOOD AND EXERCISE RECORD

Maintenance   Calories Expended

Calories_____   Per Minute of Exercise_____

Date_____   Minutes of Exercise_____

Breakfast

Lunch

Dinner

Snacks throughout the day

Total Calories Consumed _____

Less Exercise Calories

   Expended   _____

   Net   _____

   + or − Calories Over

   or Under Maintenance   _____

Weekly Calorie Balance _____ − 3,500 Calories = _____ Pound Change

(Total your daily calorie balance for 7 days and predict weight change.)

EXERCISE

When people come to me for diet advice, I always tell them that diet (by which I mean the food they eat) is only 50 percent of the weight control/fitness equation. The other half is exercise. Eating provides the motivation to exercise and exercising motivates you to eat well. Many people make the mistake of doing only one or the other, making their goal harder to reach.

Exercise also helps you lose *fat* instead of muscle. Since muscle burns a high percentage of our calorie requirement, we don't want to get rid of it!

A successful exercise program has the same requirements as a successful diet program. It must be enjoyable; it must fit into your busy life; and it must help you accomplish your goals. Consider these a little more closely:

It must be enjoyable: The food you eat must please your palate and the exercise you choose must be fun if you are going to look forward to it on a regular basis. If you like being outdoors, then choose an activity such as walking, jogging, or bicycling—and make it regular. If you prefer being indoors, or are restricted by the weather, then choose an exercise such as low-impact aerobic dance, swimming, or walking or jogging indoors. Or if you prefer exercising alone, at home, indoors, why not try a stationary bike? It is good to have two or three exercise routines—that is, cross-training. When you find an exercise that you like, write it into your schedule. Make it a priority, and it will support your goal for losing fat. Staying with it—that is the key to long-term weight management. Enjoyment makes you more likely to stay with it.

It must be convenient: Busy people are generally juggling many things—families, careers, social lives. Adding exercise to the list may be difficult to manage, but it's rewarding. A workout schedule and routine should be *convenient* so that it is more likely to be carried out. Schedule exercise the way you would any other appointment, and keep it. Choose an exercise class that's convenient enough for you to fit into your daily schedule. Choose swimming only if you have *easy* access to a swimming pool. Many people choose walking because it is generally convenient. Whether you are at home or away from home, you can always put your shoes on and walk or jog . . . or walk/jog! It's good to schedule your exercise at the same time each day—a morning, noon, or after-work schedule—this helps maintain your routine. Remember, it must be regular, it must be scheduled.

It must work: If your objective is to lose fat, then choose a calorie level, dietary fat level, and an exercise regime that will accomplish this goal. There is no such thing as "spot reducing" to get rid of fat in certain areas of the body. Although muscle building can be directed to specific muscle groups, fat losing is a different process, and happens generally from all parts of the body. Some of this is genetic and related to the body type you have. In addition, upper body fat is more easily mobilized, or used for energy than lower body fat—another reason that women, who tend to store fat in the lower body, tend to lose weight on their hips more slowly. To lose fat, *aerobic* exercise with the right amount of calories is the answer.

The chart that follows lists the energy cost of activities per minute, per pound of body weight. To determine your calorie expenditure during exercise, simply multiply your weight times the number of minutes you sustained your workout. For example, at a weight of 160, a pace of 20 minutes per mile, a 45-minute walk (.032 calories per minute) would be calculated as follows:

.032 × 160 pounds × 45 minutes = 230.4 calories

Energy Expenditure During Activities

ACTIVITY	ENERGY EXPENDITURE (calories/min./pound body weight)
Basketball	0.064
Canoeing	
Leisure	0.018
Racing*	0.045
Dancing	
Ballroom	0.023
Aerobic*	0.077
Football	0.060
Golf	0.041
(walking plus carrying bag)	
Running	
9 min./mile*	0.086
8 min./mile*	0.100
7 min./mile*	0.109
6 min./mile*	0.127
Swimming	
Backstroke*	0.077
Breaststroke*	0.073
Crawl, fast*	0.073
Crawl, slow*	0.059
Tennis (singles)	0.050
Volleyball	0.022
Walking (horizontal)	
16 min./mile*	0.036
20 min./mile*	0.032

* Aerobic forms of exercise.
Chart adapted from the American College of Sports Medicine, Guidelines for Exercise Testing and Prescription.

Aerobic Exercise

This is the kind of exercise that burns the most fat. It is called aerobic because it uses oxygen while it burns calories. Aerobic exercise is any activity that puts a moderate demand on your heart, blood vessels, lungs, and muscles for a relatively continuous time (twenty to thirty minutes or longer). This helps to achieve cardiovascular fitness while burning fat. Exercises that are considered aerobic include the following: brisk walking, jogging, swimming, cycling, aerobic dance, stair climbing, rowing. Depending on your size and the intensity of your exercise session, you will burn 5 to 10 calories per minute doing one of these exercises.

Exercising every two or three days is a good start, with a goal of three to six days a week. To improve cardiovascular fitness, a minimum of three times per week and preferably four is needed. If you are having a hard time fitting exercise into your schedule, remember that a walk around the block twice a week is better than no walk at all, even if the long-term goal is to walk six days a week for thirty minutes. You don't have to be a marathoner. A study published in the November 1989 *Journal of American Medical Association* conducted by the Institute for Aerobics Research and Cooper Clinic tracked the fitness and health of 13,000 men and women over an eight-year period, and found that even moderate exercise can lead to increase in longevity—in fact, the greatest health benefit was gained by sedentary individuals who began very light, moderate exercise, as in walking briskly for a half hour several days a week. Start somewhere, even if it's only for ten minutes a day.

Studies show that exercising six days a week may be better than only three or four, even when total calories expended are equal. Frequent exercise produces body steroids that stimulate fat cells to burn fat. According to the American College of Sports Medicine's "Position Stand on Proper and Improper Weight Loss Programs," significant changes in body fat can be achieved when a 500-calorie restriction is combined with three to five days of exercise, with each session burning 300 to 500 calories. More exercise can mean more injuries, so be sure to build your routine slowly. To gain other benefits, such as decreased blood pressure and increased HDL cholesterol, burning 1,000 calories per week, ideally in four to five sessions over the course of a week is suggested.*

For those with a lot of weight to lose, walking, swimming, or stationary biking are preferred over running, aerobic dance, or jumping rope. Once a normal weight range is achieved, aerobic exercise three to four times per week is probably sufficient to maintain weight. A rule of thumb is to *work toward* exercising to the degree that you will burn around *1,800 calories per week*, or 300 calories per session, six days a week—in order to lose body fat. And what happens if you stop exercising for two weeks? Is it necessary to start all over? Per-

* Falco, J.M., O'Dorisio, T.M., and Cataland, S., "Improvement of High Density Lipoprotein Cholesterol levels," *Journal of American Medical Association*, Vol. 247 (1982): 37–40.

haps you will need to ease into your routine, but the longer you have been exercising, the faster you'll regain your fitness level.

How Hard Should You Exercise?

The intensity of exercise is the most critical factor for aerobic conditioning and fat burning. Exercise must be strenuous enough to increase the heart rate to between 70 to 80 percent of your maximum heart rate, as determined by a standard maximum heart rate of 220 beats per minute, and your age. Your target heart-rate zone is the heart rate at which you will get the most benefits from exercise. Check the chart below that lists the Maximum Exercise Heart Rate and Target Zones for both a full minute and for ten-second intervals, for various ages.

Maximum Exercise Heart Rate and Target Zones

AGE	M.E.H.R.	60%–80% BEATS PER MINUTE	MAXIMUM BEATS PER 10 SECONDS
20	200	120–160	20–26
25	195	117–156	20–26
30	190	114–152	19–25
35	185	111–148	19–25
40	180	108–144	21–26
45	175	105–140	18–23
50	170	102–136	17–23
55	165	99–132	17–22
60	160	96–128	16–21
65	155	93–124	16–21
70	150	90–120	15–20
75	145	87–116	15–19
80	140	84–112	14–19

Keep in mind that the target zone changes with age. Be aware also that the amount of exercise it takes to put you in your target zone changes with your fitness level. As you get into better shape, your heart rate will be lower for the same amount of exercise. So then you'll have to work harder to get it higher and, in the process, achieve even greater fitness. If you have been sedentary, you can even begin to see an improvement in your fitness level if you exercise at 40 to 50 percent of your heart rate reserve (as opposed to 70 to 85 percent listed in the chart). If you are on blood pressure medication, or a medication for your heart, your heart rate may not rise, and these target heart-rate zones do not apply to you. Check with your doctor to determine the appropriate intensity level of exercise.

It is a good idea to take your pulse before, during, and right after exercise. There are many good pulse monitors on the market today, but if you don't have one, you can take your own pulse, by either pressing against your carotid artery (under your jaw to your collarbone down either side of your neck) or on the inside of your wrist below the bone of your thumb. Be careful not to press too hard—this may cause your heart rate to decrease. Using a second hand on your watch or a digital readout of seconds, count the number of times your heart beats in ten seconds, beginning with zero.

Notice that when you are below your target heart-rate zone, you are not breathing very deeply, and it seems too easy—you may not be getting all the benefits of aerobic exercise, unless you are at a very low fitness level. When you are above your zone, your face may be flushed and you may be overdoing it. When you are in your target zone, you will generally be exercising hard enough to sweat. That's great! You are burning up calories through the production of heat. It may take a while before you start sweating during each exercise session. That's fine, too. Don't rush to your target zone too quickly.

And always remember to warm up and cool down before and after a workout. Warm up by performing your activity *slowly* for three to five minutes, then do slow, gentle stretches with your legs, arms, and torso. Avoid bouncing, as a sudden movement in a cold muscle may cause an injury. Slowly increase your exercise intensity until you reach your target heart rate.

"Cooling down" after exercise means simply to "keep moving." If you stop suddenly after exercise, blood pools in the legs, decreasing blood supply to the brain, which could cause you to faint, particularly if you have been sedentary for a long time. Check your heart rate again after you have cooled down. A goal is to have your heart rate below one hundred beats per minute before you end your cool-down portion of exercise. As you become more physically fit, your heart rate will return to normal more quickly.

How Long Should You Exercise?

The *time* spent exercising is just as important as the *intensity*, so if you're just starting out, exercise at a slower pace for a longer period of time. Begin at your current level of capability, and work toward a thirty- to forty-five-minute session. Research shows that burning at least 300 calories per exercise session is necessary to affect body fat significantly. This could be accomplished by a three-mile walk or jog, or forty-five minutes on the stationary bike. Although it is best for the exercise to be a continuous session, discontinuous exercise also provides a benefit. For example, a fifteen-minute bike ride to work in the morning and a fifteen-minute bike ride home in the evening will make you feel good and will help improve aerobic condition, although not as much as an uninterrupted thirty-minute bike ride.

Start-and-stop exercises, such as tennis, basketball, and racquetball, must be engaged in for longer periods of time to produce *cardiovascular* benefits. If you play hard enough, have some basic skills in the game, and play with an opponent of similar skill, you will generally get benefit from forty to sixty minutes of play, depending on the intensity. Certain sports, such as recreational softball, bowling, and golf cannot provide cardiovascular fitness benefits no matter how long they are played, because their intensity level is too low. However, these are still good recreational activities, and we cannot overlook the value of the relaxation, as well as the minor increase in calorie expenditure and local muscular development.

You should check with your doctor before you begin any exercise program, particularly if you have been inactive. If this is the case, you should start slowly, for about ten to twenty minutes, two to three times per week. As you get into better shape, you can gradually increase the exercise time of each session as well as the number of times you exercise each week.

Measuring Progress with Body Composition

The bathroom scale may tell you the number of pounds you have lost, but a true measure of success is making sure that you are losing fat, not muscle. By choosing the right balance of calories and exercise, you can not only lose pounds but get that lean and fit look, much more attractive than the "skinny" look.

There are several methods of measuring body composition, including measuring fat with calipers (sometimes called the "pinch test") and the underwater weighing method (most accurate), which compares your land weight to your water weight, based on the principle that muscle is more dense than fat and therefore a heavier underwater weight means a lower body fat. Although this method is most accurate, it is not always practical, since it requires dunking an individual in a tank of water. Another method is the bioelectrical impedance testing. Electrodes are hooked up to the hands and feet, and a very slight electrical current is passed from one set of electrodes to the other (you don't feel the current). The resistance measured is used along with height, weight, and sex to calculate the body fat to lean ratio. If you have access to any of these methods, by all means measure your body fat before you get started and then repeat at six-week intervals. Don't be discouraged if the scale doesn't show a weight change. It is possible to gain muscle as you lose fat. But don't fool yourself, either. Muscle is generally gained more slowly than fat is lost. A typical walking, jogging, biking, or dancing program as we have recommended may result in a lean mass increase of about one pound a month, perhaps more in a person who has been sedentary. Those who engage in serious weight training may gain up to two to three pounds of muscle per month, particularly if there is no calorie restriction.

The real test, of course, is how you feel, how you look, and how your clothes fit—and as you begin to firm up and lose fat, you're bound to feel great!

CHAPTER · 8

FAST-FOOD RATINGS

RATING THE FAST FOODS

Nutrition and fast food for many years seemed to be at opposite ends of the table. If you had healthy foods and nutritious meals, it usually required quite a bit of preparation time. If you chose a "heat and eat" or "cheat and eat" lifestyle and used convenience foods, it was a sacrifice of good nutrition. Now that healthy eating is becoming a more mainstream concept, food manufacturers are giving consumers what they want as they make fast and processed foods—frozen dinners, salad dressings, canned soups—more healthy. New products that speed along a home-cooked meal have also appeared on the market—pizza crusts, spaghetti sauce, muffin mixes. Even fast-food chains are responding to our request for low-fat meals as they offer chili, broiled chicken sandwiches, fat-free muffins, salads, even carrot sticks—all interesting low-fat alternatives to double cheeseburgers. At last, it is possible to get healthy, fast, and tasty all in the same fast-lane meal.

Not all new foods are changing for the better, of course, but some are. It is the purpose of this chapter to show you which of the fast foods live up to the nutritional claims on their packages and which actually sabotage our efforts to eat a better diet. In this chapter, we will look at frozen foods, including breakfast items, single-item snacks, lunches, and dinners. Then we'll take a look at the deli and fresh-refrigerated foods, such as light sandwich meats, premixed tuna salad, potato salad, and specialty pasta items. We will examine new foods available at the supermarket, including produce items, canned goods, salad dressings, boxed breads, and boxed meals (from macaroni and cheese to Hamburger Helper to pasta salad mixes). And, of course, we will rate the best and the worst of fast-food restaurant fare.

FROZEN FOODS

Frozen foods can be a healthy part of your Fast-Food Diet, thanks to changes manufacturers have made since the days of the "TV dinners" that came in those aluminum trays. Now, there are many frozen dinners that meet the healthy criteria of low calories, less than 30 percent fat, less than 1,000 milligrams of sodium, and one-third the U.S. recommended daily allowance for certain vitamins and minerals, as well as protein.

One of the most important things frozen foods do for the health-conscious, weight-conscious shopper is to say no for you, since they come in preset portions. This is one of the principal reasons for the popularity of weight-loss centers where the meals with preset portions must be purchased and eaten. These meals leave no room for a little extra oil, or a topping of cheese that doesn't belong, not to mention larger portions and extra bites. But why hassle with diet-center food when the same low-calorie, low-fat, portion-controlled frozen dinners are available in the frozen-food section of your supermarket? Compare the cost: most frozen entrées are under five dollars, with an average cost of about three dollars. This may be more economical than home cooking when you figure in the time factor, and it's an inexpensive alternative to dining out.

Remember, though, that even the best of these frozen dishes does not make a completely balanced meal. Like the commercial fast foods, most are low in calcium, vitamins A and C, and fiber. Consequently, I recommend that you supplement them with a salad or another vegetable side dish, whole-grain bread or roll, low-fat dairy, and/or a piece of fresh fruit. A small salad, a slice of bread, and an eight-ounce glass of nonfat milk add only 300 calories. Know your calorie goal for the day. If you are a five-foot two-inch woman and your daily goal is 800 calories, you will want to emphasize vegetables (lower in calories) as opposed to entrées. If, on the other hand, you are a five-foot eight-inch-tall woman and expend 300 calories a day in exercise, you can lose weight on 1,500 calories, in which case you may be able to afford the extra calories that come with the added nutrients. In general, choose frozen meals that contain 300 calories or less and are no more than 30 percent fat (10 grams or less).

The charts that follow rate dozens of frozen foods (pages 154–156). Since hundreds of new items are introduced each year (and some of your favorites may be taken off the market), you may want to learn to calculate the percentage of calories from fat for yourself to determine whether you are within the 30 percent fat limit. Simply multiply the number of fat grams times nine and divide this figure by the number of total calories. For example, a 250-calorie meal of Healthy Choice lasagna with meat sauce lists 4 grams of fat. Each of the 4 fat grams provide 9 calories, for a total of 36 calories from fat. Divide the 36 by 250 and you get 0.144, or about 14 percent fat, well within the limit.

If cholesterol is not listed, just remember that a *three-ounce* serving of red meat or chicken provides about *25 percent* of the 300 milligrams of cholesterol per day suggested in the National Cholesterol Education Program Guidelines. White fish has less, shellfish has more, and vegetables have none, unless cheese is added. (See Appendix B for cholesterol content of common foods.)

For a real treat, make your own frozen entrées for days when you don't feel like cooking from scratch. These meals may be less expensive, and you will have full control over what goes into them. Items that freeze nicely include the following: fish, chicken, pizza (before baking), turkey burgers, corn chowder soup, pasta sauce, and ratatouille. (See complete list on page 169.)

DELI AND FRESH-REFRIGERATED FOODS

The deli caters to busy people who have a taste for more than just burgers and fries, for everyday needs or for parties. (See Party Snacks, Chapter 15, to discover a new way of purchasing food for elegant or casual dining with less work and time.) But buyer beware, for without careful scrutiny, it's also easy to end up with a high-fat meal.

One problem with deli foods, unlike fast-food franchise style or frozen dinners, is that there is no consistency. Recipes vary drastically from cook to cook, even within the same deli. But, on the other hand, you have the advantage of seeing what you are buying. So follow these guidelines and refer to the ratings of *typical* deli foods to make your decision:

Limit portions: If you are eating an item for lunch or dinner that is prepared with a significant amount of fat (and your eye will tell you), limit the portion size to a half cup or two to four ounces. This includes dinner entrées such as kung pao chicken (seasoned chicken with peanuts); pasta with sauce; as well as typical sandwich fillings, tuna salad, crab salad, and calamari (squid) salad. Here, you are getting protein and fat, and, in order to make it a healthy choice, you must balance out the ratio of carbohydrate to fat and protein by adding an unbuttered whole-grain or sourdough roll and an apple or an orange.

Add food to dilute fat: If you are using the deli item at home and have the opportunity to "fix" it, you can do so quickly by adding more starch and vegetables to the fatty mixture. For example, add potatoes or vegetables (onions, celery, chopped carrots) to potato salad, assorted vegetables and extra pasta to pasta dishes, carrots or cucumber to three bean salad.

Choose the right sauce: If you are buying an item to cook or reheat at home, such as marinated meat, chicken, or fish, choose one in an oil rather than cream-based sauce, and add no additional fat when cooking. If you broil or grill marinated foods, most of the fat drips off—so it usually is fairly low-fat. Lamb or chicken brochettes help to control portion sizes. On your own, limit portion size to three to four ounces of animal protein, and again, balance out the ratio of carbohydrate to fat by adding a vegetable, potato, rice, or a bread.

Supplement with vegetables: Make sure your meal includes vegetables to add vitamins, minerals, and fiber. Many delis also carry produce, in which case, simply pick up a cucumber, a tomato, or a few carrots. Wash, slice and eat. If your deli has a salad bar, use it. Just make a commitment to getting the vegetables back into your dinner.

Supermarket Deli Foods

FOODS	PORTION SIZE	FAT (G)	CALORIES
Apple turnovers	1 each	4.6	85
Bologna			
Beef	1 slice	6.8	75
Turkey	1 slice	4.5	60
Carrot-raisin salad	½ cup	6	150
Cheeses:			
American, Cheddar, Muenster	1 oz.	9.5	115
Chicken			
Fried	1 breast	17.4	435
Baked	1 breast	11.7	330
Salad	1 cup	36	500
Chopped liver	1 cup	8	220
Coleslaw	1 cup	17	175
Crab salad	3½ oz.	8.5	145
Egg salad	½ cup	33	364
Fruit salad	1 cup	1	125

FOODS	PORTION SIZE	FAT (G)	CALORIES
Ham	1 oz.	1.2	34
Honeyloaf	1 oz.	33	1.2
Salad	1 oz.	4.3	60
Slices	1 oz.	2.9	50
Herring—pickled	3½ oz.	15.3	225
Lox	1 oz.	2.2	52
Macaroni and beef	1 cup	8	225
Macaroni salad	1 cup	14	240
Pizza			
Pepperoni	1 slice	11.5	305
Sausage	1 slice	14.2	340
Potato salad	1 cup	23.2	360
Rigatoni, salami, beef	1 slice	4.8	60
Sandwiches			
Bacon, lettuce, tomato, mayo on white		15.6	280
Corned beef on rye		8.4	230
Chicken salad on white		9	245
Egg salad on white		12.4	280
Peanut butter and jelly on whole wheat		15.4	385
Roast beef and mayo on white		22.7	330
Tuna salad on white		14.3	280
Turkey on whole wheat with mustard		5.8	260
Sausage, pork or beef	1 link	23	265
Tuna salad	½ cup	11	175

GETTING THE MOST FROM CONVENIENCE FOODS

There are many new convenience foods on the market that make it easy to eat more healthfully. But while some are truly good choices, others will only increase the fat and calorie content of your diets. I have rated these foods—produce, sandwich meats, bottled spaghetti sauces, boxed mixes of muffins, macaroni and cheese, even pasta salad mixes—to provide you with a guide to the world of fast convenient food. (See pages 150–153.)

You must watch out for fat and sodium when buying convenience foods. When you use convenience foods that are ready to eat or that only need heating, you have little control over the amount of fat and sodium. You may find that what you are looking for is available in a reduced-calorie, lower fat, or reduced-sodium form. Note that lower sodium versions of products are not necessarily low in fat—soups, for example. Also be aware that products designed to be lower in fat may sometimes be higher in sodium or cholesterol, or both. For example, a tablespoon of one brand of reduced-calorie French dressing contains 7 grams less fat but 115 milligrams *more* sodium than the same amount of regular French dressing. Compared with an all-beef hot dog, a chicken hot dog has 4 grams less fat, and 115 milligrams *more* sodium and 23 milligrams *more* cholesterol. My rating system takes all of these variables into account.

You do have more control over partially prepared mixes that call for added ingredients such as salt, margarine, butter, or milk. For example, by using half as much margarine called for on a box mix of macaroni and cheese, and using low-fat milk, you can save 8 grams of fat per serving (almost 2 teaspoons, or 100 calories).

FAST-FOOD RESTAURANTS

Fast foods have been singled out as a symbol of what is wrong with nutrition in the United States today. But, the main problem with most fast-food meals is the same as with a steak dinner in the finest restaurant: it is not nutritionally balanced. They provide too many calories and too much fat, particularly saturated fat.

Still, I have promised that eating well need not be an all-or-nothing proposition. My clients who like to eat at fast-food restaurants are often surprised to hear me say, "We can work it into your plan." Although every item available at a fast-food restaurant is not a nutritional virtue, they are responding to criticism that they are nutritional nightmares. Chains are broadening their menus, so among the burgers and fries are lower-fat alternatives, such as the grilled chicken sandwiches, salads, baked potatoes, chili, low-fat salad dressing, fruit juices, low-fat or skim milk and whole-grain buns.

Menu Advancements

McDonald's: In addition to adding new products to the menu, McDonald's has taken measures to improve the nutritional value of its existing menu items. Menu enhancements include switching to 100% vegetable oil for preparing french fries, as well as all their fried sandwiches, Chicken McNuggets, and hot pie desserts. (Still, they *are* fried.) They have also reduced the amount of sodium in their hotcakes, pickles, and breakfast sausage. They offer low-fat frozen yogurt instead of soft serve. Their breakfast menu has been expanded with no-fat, no-cholesterol apple bran muffins and whole-grain cereals. They are now serving only low-fat milk shakes. They have replaced 2% milk with 1% low-fat milk, and added calcium to their sandwich buns: Ready-to-eat salads are available. Low-oil versions of sandwich sauces with 50 percent less fat will be replacing old stand-bys. Nutrition information is available at each restaurant.

Wendy's: Long recognized as a leader in providing options and choices to its customers, Wendy's was among the first to offer an extensive salad bar, as well as baked potatoes and, my favorite, chili. Their new SuperBar offers a hot and cold food buffet which includes pasta with several sauces—I suggest the tomato based spaghetti sauce. The expanded salad bar includes fresh fruit as well as fresh vegetables. New menu choices include a grilled chicken sandwich made with skinless, boneless breast of chicken topped with fresh lettuce and tomato. (Honey mustard sauce is optional.) At the time of this writing, they are testing a lower-fat Frosty Dairy Dessert and a new low-fat frozen yogurt. Nutrition information is now available at each restaurant.

Hardee's: Also a leader in broadening the fast-food offerings, Hardee's now offers prepackaged salads and a grilled chicken sandwich which is nonbreaded and nonfried. They offer reduced calorie mayonnaise for sandwiches with mayonnaise. They were the very first to cook french fries and all other fried products in all-vegetable oil. They have recently added pancakes to their breakfast menu, and are testing products like their Lean-1, a ¼-pound hamburger, which they claim will have the lowest total fat that is being offered as a standard menu item among the "burger giants."

Jack in the Box: Take-out salads including chef, taco, and side-salad have long been offered at Jack in the Box. They offer a low-calorie French salad dressing. Their sesame bread sticks are a nice accompaniment. They were among the other fast-food restaurants in switching to all-vegetable oil. Their nutritional pride is their chicken fajita pita, which is available with or without the cheese. (They are one of the biggest users of pita bread in the country.) They also offer a grilled chicken fillet (a boneless, skinless chicken breast on a whole-wheat bun). They offer low-fat milk. Nutritional information is available at each restaurant.

General Fast-Food Rules

Here are some simple and healthy "eat and run" rules for getting the most (healthwise) out of a fast-food restaurant.

Keep it plain and simple: If you want to keep the calories under 500 and the fat less than 30 percent, you can do it by ordering a simple hamburger, taco, or chicken or roast beef sandwich and a diet drink, iced tea, or better yet, low-fat milk or orange juice. If a plain side salad or a baked potato is offered, you may want to choose that option. Avoid extra-crispy chicken.

The smallest burger offered at each of the five major fast-food restaurants *has always been* the lowest-fat option. The chart below lists the varying sizes and fat content of a few hamburger patties:

RESTAURANT	WEIGHT OF SMALLEST BURGER (OUNCES)	FAT (G)
McDonald's	1.14	6
Wendy's	2.6	12
Roy Rogers	2.6	18
Hardee's	1.13	6.9
Burger King	1.39	8.9

Of course, the bigger the burger, the more fat. If you order the deluxe burgers, you are likely to go over your limit.* The Burger King Whopper contains 36 grams of fat, Wendy's Classic Cheeseburger has 39 grams of fat, McDonald's Quarter Pounder, 21, with their Big Mac at 32 grams.

There is a difference of 18 to 22 grams of fat or roughly 650 calories, between the plain hamburger and the deluxe burger. That's a whole meal's worth of calories. Why not keep it simple? Cut out the extras. Secret sauce, tartar sauce, or mayonnaise add about 50 calories per tablespoon, mostly fat calories. Avoid ordering items with *extra* cheese, bacon, or sausage. Steer away from breaded and fried fish or chicken unless you feel okay about removing the skin.

* Calculate your fat limit in grams by multiplying your daily calorie goal by 30 percent (.30, then dividing by 9. For example, if 30 percent of 1,500 calories was fat, that would be 450 fat calories, or 50 grams of fat:

1500 × .30 = 450

450 ÷ 9 = 50 grams

French fries versus baked potato: It was international news when the major fast-food restaurants switched to all vegetable oil. That's a step in the right direction, but remember that even the smallest order of fries adds about 12 grams of fat. Those restaurants who cook their fries in all vegetable oil at the date of this writing include Hardee's, Wendy's, and Burger King. This switch from one fat to the other improves the *kind of fat,* it does not decrease the total fat or calories.

The baked potatoes offered at several places are good alternatives to the fries, when eaten with minimal added fat. Here's how they stack up:

	FAT (G)	CALORIES
Baked potato, plain	0	140
Baked potato w/2 tbsp. sour cream and chives	5	200
Baked potato w/4 oz. cheese	34	590
Regular fries	12	220
Large fries	16	320

Salads as saviors? Fast foods tend to be low in fiber. Salad bars can help compensate for this lack. They also add vitamin C and beta carotene. Of the five major fast-food restaurants, McDonald's, Burger King, Wendy's, Hardee's, and Roy Rogers offer at least one salad, some offer two or three. Wendy's has been a leader with a salad bar in every restaurant, with 60 percent of its restaurants offering a "super salad bar," that includes more salads and a few hot foods. Roy Rogers also offers a salad bar. Those salads I tested were made with fresh ingredients and were quite acceptable, although I would rather see more vegetables and less meat and cheese. Each bar has a low-calorie salad dressing.

Don't assume that a fast-food salad is necessarily better than a burger. The way the salad is prepared or what you put on it may make it just as high in fat as the burgers and fries. Refer to Chapters 11 and 12 on lunches and salads for fat and calories savings from salad makeovers. Here are a few examples of popular fast-food salads.

	FAT (G)	CALORIES
Wendy's Taco Salad	37	660
Wendy's Chef Salad (no dressing)	9	180
McDonald's Side Salad	3	60
McDonald's Chef Salad	13	230
Taco Bell Taco Salad with salsa and shell	61	941
Hardee's Chicken 'n' Pasta Salad	3	230
Hardee's Chef Salad	15	240

NOTE: All creamy dressings are 100 calories per ladle; diet dressings vary.

McDonald's newly packaged carrot and celery sticks offer an excellent new choice.

Beverage options exist: Shakes provide between 300 and 500 calories and around 10 grams of fat. This is too many if you are trying to limit calories. They do provide a fairly good calcium source—about 320 milligrams per twelve-ounce shake, but at the expense of adding fat. McDonald's has introduced a lower-fat milk-shake mix. Wendy's is planning to reduce the fat in their Frosty. Still, the plain low-fat milk provides a good dose of calcium (one cup has close to 300 milligrams of calcium) and has two-thirds less calories than the shake.

Desserts are improving, too: Soft-serve ice cream cones are an option, at 170 to 185 calories and 5 grams of fat for a three-ounce cone—better than Dairy Queen's Hot Fudge Brownie Delight at 570 calories and 22 grams of fat. Look for the new frozen yogurt offerings, or orange sherbet, or have a piece of fruit when you return to your home or office. Skip fried fruit pies, which are 250 to 400 calories each, with 14 grams of fat, or 50 percent of calories. Some cookies, such as the McDonaldland animal cracker variety, are 300 calories a box, and 12 grams of fat, or 32 percent of calories, perhaps reasonable if you shared them with someone. But on top of a meal, dessert may add too many calories.

Work toward daily balance: If you ate too much at lunch, consider the meal to be your main meal of the day and go for a light low-fat dinner.

Add a salad, or a bowl of broccoli at dinner; have an apple or banana later.

Breakfast alternatives: The breakfast business at fast-food restaurants has increased dramatically. Although you can hold the egg sandwich in one hand while you drive with the other, this is not the best way to start a busy day. I suggest the English muffins with light margarine, jam, and orange juice or low-fat milk. McDonald's has added cereal to its breakfast offering, as well as a fat-free apple-bran muffin. I look forward to these alternatives to the egg, sausage, pancakes, and Danish.

Nutrition information about the restaurant's foods is often available for the asking. By careful discrimination, you can come a lot closer to the recommended dietary guidelines, even if you can't always meet them. Check the chart in this chapter to see how all your fast-food choices rate in nutrition, according to my scale.

ARBY'S

	Rating	Calories	Fat (g)	Saturated Fat (g)	Cholesterol (mg)	Sodium (mg)	Fiber (g)
Baked Potato, Plain	10	290	1	—	0	12	>1.5
Baked Potato, Superstuffed, Broccoli & Cheddar	8	541	22	—	24	475	>1.5
Baked Potato, Superstuffed, Deluxe	6	648	38	—	72	475	>1.5
Baked Potato, Superstuffed, Mushroom & Cheese	5	506	22	—	21	635	>1.5
Chicken Breast, Roasted*	5	254	7	—	196	930	<1.5
Hot Ham 'n Cheese Sandwich	5	353	13	—	50	1655	<1.5
French Dip Roast Beef Sandwich*	5	386	12	—	55	1111	<1.5
Junior Roast Beef*	4	218	8	—	20	345	<1.5
Arby's Sub (no dressing)	4	484	16	—	58	1354	<1.5
Turkey Deluxe*	4	375	17	—	39	850	<1.5
Super Roast Beef	4	501	22	—	40	800	<1.5
King Roast Beef	4	467	19	—	49	765	<1.5
Baked Potato, Superstuffed, Taco	4	619	27	—	145	1065	>1.5
Chicken Salad Sandwich	4	386	20	—	30	630	<1.5
French Fries*	4	211	8	—	6	30	<1.5
Mushroom & Swiss Croissant	4	340	18	—	60	630	<1.5
Roast Beef Deluxe	4	486	23	—	59	1288	<1.5
Regular Roast Beef	4	353	15	—	39	590	<1.5
Ham & Swiss Croissant	4	330	15	—	70	995	<1.5
Bacon & Egg Croissant	4	420	25	—	440	550	<1.5
Chicken Breast Sandwich	3	592	27	—	57	1340	<1.5
Chicken Club Sandwich	3	621	32	—	108	1300	<1.5

ARBY'S (continued)

	Rating	Calories	Fat (g)	Saturated Fat (g)	Cholesterol (mg)	Sodium (mg)	Fiber (g)
Butter Croissant*	3	220	**10**	—	50	225	<1.5
Potato Cakes*	3	201	**14**	—	13	425	<1.5
Bac'n Cheddar Deluxe Roast Beef*	3	561	**34**	—	78	**1385**	<1.5
Apple Turnover*†	3	310	**21**	—	NA	240	<1.5
Sausage & Egg Croissant*	3	499	**33**	—	**645**	**705**	<1.5
Beef 'n Cheddar	3	490	**21**	—	51	**1520**	<1.5
Blueberry Turnover*†	2	340	**20**	—	NA	255	<1.5
Cherry Turnover*†	2	320	**20**	—	NA	254	<1.5
Chicken Salad Croissant*	2	460	**36**	—	**111**	**725**	<1.5

* LOSES ADDITIONAL POINTS DUE TO LOW VITAMIN AND MINERAL CONTENT.

† LOSES ADDITIONAL POINT DUE TO HIGH SUGAR CONTENT.

NOTE: BOLDFACE NUMBERS INDICATE NUTRITIONAL FACTOR THAT DETRACTS FROM FOOD'S NUTRITIONAL VALUE (see the note on page 22).

ARTHUR TREACHER'S

	Rating	Calories	Fat (g)	Saturated Fat (g)	Cholesterol (mg)	Sodium (mg)	Fiber (g)
Coleslaw	7	123	**8**	1	7	266	<1.5
Fish Sandwich*	5	440	**24**	4	42	**836**	<1.5
Chicken Sandwich*	5	413	**19**	3	3	**708**	<1.5
Chips (French Fries)*	5	276	**13**	2	1	39	<1.5
Fish, Fried, 2 pieces*	5	355	**20**	3	56	450	<1.5
Chicken, Fried*	5	369	**22**	4	65	495	<1.5
Lemon Luv (Fried Pie)*†	4	276	**14**	2	1	314	<1.5
Shrimp, Fried*	4	381	**24**	3	**93**	538	<1.5
Chowder*	3	112	**5**	**2**	9	**835**	<1.5
Krunch Pup (Batter-fried Hot Dog)*	3	203	**15**	4	25	446	<1.5

* LOSES ADDITIONAL POINTS DUE TO LOW VITAMIN AND MINERAL CONTENT.

† LOSES ADDITIONAL POINT DUE TO HIGH SUGAR CONTENT.

NOTE: BOLDFACE NUMBERS INDICATE NUTRITIONAL FACTOR THAT DETRACTS FROM FOOD'S NUTRITIONAL VALUE (see the note on page 22).

BURGER KING

	Rating	Calories	Fat (g)	Saturated Fat (g)	Cholesterol (mg)	Sodium (mg)	Fiber (g)
Bagel*	7	272	6	1	29	438	<1.5
Side Salad w/1 tbsp. reduced-cal light Italian dressing	7	68	4.5	0.8	1	218	>1.5
Chunky Chicken Salad w/1 tbsp. reduced-cal light Italian dressing	7	185	8.5	1.8	50	634	>1.5
Garden Salad w/1 tbsp. reduced-cal light Italian dressing	6	138	9.5	3.8	16	316	>1.5
French Toast Sticks w/Burger King A.M. Express Dip*†	6	622	32	5	80	555	>1.5
Broiler Chicken Sandwich* (on oat-bran bun)	6	379	18	3	53	764	>1.5
Ocean Catch Fish Filet* (on oat-bran bun)	6	495	25	4	57	879	>1.5
Chicken Tenders, 6 pieces*	5	236	13	3	46	541	<1.5
Bagel w/Cream Cheese*	5	370	16	6	58	523	<1.5
Onion Rings, regular*	5	302	17	4	3	559	<1.5
Hash Browns*	5	213	12	3	3	318	<1.5
Hamburger*	5	272	11	4	37	505	<1.5
Croissant*	5	180	10	2	4	285	<1.5
Biscuit*	5	332	17	3	2	754	<1.5
Chief Salad w/1 tbsp. reduced-cal light Italian dressing	4	221	13.5	4.8	104	759	>1.5
Bagel Sandwich w/Ham, Egg, & Cheese	4	438	17	6	266	1114	<1.5
Hamburger Deluxe*	4	344	19	6	43	496	<1.5
French Fries, regular*	4	341	20	10	21	241	<1.5
Scrambled Egg Platter (eggs, croissant, hash browns)	4	549	34	9	365	893	<1.5
Whopper	3	614	36	12	90	865	<1.5
Mushroom Swiss Double Cheeseburger	3	473	27	12	95	746	<1.5
Bagel Sandwich w/Egg, & Cheese*	3	407	16	5	247	759	<1.5
Biscuit w/Bacon*	3	378	20	5	8	867	<1.5
Bagel Sandwich w/Bacon, Egg & Cheese*	3	453	20	7	252	872	<1.5
Biscuit w/Bacon & Egg*	3	467	27	7	213	1033	<1.5
Biscuit w/Sausage*	3	478	29	8	33	1007	<1.5
Apple Pie*†	3	311	14	4	4	412	<1.5
Whopper w/Cheese	3	706	44	16	115	1177	<1.5
Bacon Double Cheeseburger	3	515	31	14	105	748	<1.5
Barbecue Bacon Double Cheeseburger	3	536	31	14	105	795	<1.5
Biscuit w/Sausage and Egg	3	568	36	10	238	1172	<1.5
Croissan'wich w/Sausage, Egg, & Cheese	3	534	40	13	268	985	<1.5
Scrambled Egg Platter w/Bacon	3	610	39	11	373	1043	<1.5
Scrambled Egg Platter w/Sausage	3	768	53	15	412	1271	<1.5
Bacon Double Cheeseburger Deluxe	3	592	39	16	111	804	<1.5
Double Whopper	3	844	53	19	169	933	<1.5
Double Whopper w/Cheese	3	935	61	24	194	1245	<1.5
Cheeseburger*	3	318	15	7	50	661	<1.5
Double Cheeseburger	3	483	27	13	100	851	<1.5
Fish Tenders*	3	267	16	3	28	870	<1.5

BURGER KING (continued)

	Rating	Calories	Fat (g)	Saturated Fat (g)	Cholesterol (mg)	Sodium (mg)	Fiber (g)
Croissan'wich w/Egg & Cheese*	2	315	**20**	**7**	**222**	**607**	<1.5
Croissan'wich w/Bacon, Egg, & Cheese*	2	361	**24**	**8**	**227**	**719**	<1.5
Croissan'wich w/Ham, Egg, & Cheese*	2	346	**21**	**7**	**241**	**962**	<1.5
Danish (typical)*†	2	500	**36**	**23**	6	288	<1.5

* LOSES ADDITIONAL POINTS DUE TO LOW VITAMIN AND MINERAL CONTENT.

† LOSES ADDITIONAL POINT DUE TO HIGH SUGAR CONTENT.

NOTE: BOLDFACE NUMBERS INDICATE NUTRITIONAL FACTOR THAT DETRACTS FROM FOOD'S NUTRITIONAL VALUE (see the note on page 22).

CARL'S JR.

	Rating	Calories	Fat (g)	Saturated Fat (g)	Cholesterol (mg)	Sodium (mg)	Fiber (g)
Baked Potato, plain	10	167	2	—	0	6	1.5
Lite Potato*	9	250	0.3	0	0	35	>1.5
Salad, regular w/1 tbsp. low-cal Italian dressing	9	233	6.5	—	0	**785**	>1.5
Sour Cream & Chive Potato	8	350	**13**	**5**	10	140	>1.5
Broccoli and Cheese Potato	8	470	**17**	5	10	**690**	>1.5
California Roast Beef Sandwich	7	300	7	—	60	505	<1.5
Bran Muffin*†	7	220	6	0	50	300	1.5
Chicken Salad-to-Go w/1 tbsp. low-cal Italian dressing	6	229	**10.5**	**3**	83	543	<1.5
Old-Fashioned Chicken Noodle Soup*	6	80	**1**	trace	14	**605**	<1.5
Lumber Jack Mix Vegetable Soup	6	70	**3**	trace	3	**807**	<1.5
Blueberry Muffin*†	6	256	7	1	34	360	<1.5
Cheese Potato	6	550	**22**	**7**	40	**785**	>1.5
Fiesta Potato	6	550	**23**	**9**	40	**1230**	>1.5
Charbroiler Chicken Club Sandwich	6	510	**22**	2	85	**1165**	<1.5
Charbroiler Chicken Sandwich*	6	450	14	—	55	**1380**	<1.5
Danish (varieties)*†	6	300	9	3	0	550	<1.5
Hot Cakes with Syrup & Butter*†	6	480	15	—	15	530	<1.5
Garden Salad-to-Go w/1 tbsp. low-cal Italian dressing	5	69	**4.5**	1	7	147	<1.5
Chef Salad-to-Go w/1 tbsp. low-cal Italian dressing	5	203	**9.5**	3	63	**671**	<1.5
Bacon & Cheese Potato	5	650	**34**	**12**	45	**1820**	>1.5
Super Star Hamburger	5	780	**50**	4	**155**	785	<1.5
Cream of Broccoli Soup	4	140	**6**	4	22	**845**	<1.5
Happy Star Hamburger*	4	330	**13**	4	40	**670**	<1.5
French Toast Dips*	4	480	**25**	**10**	54	576	<1.5
Onion Rings*	4	330	**17**	**7**	15	75	<1.5

CARL'S JR. (continued)

	Rating	Calories	Fat (g)	Saturated Fat (g)	Cholesterol (mg)	Sodium (mg)	Fiber (g)
Fillet of Fish Sandwich, fried	4	570	**27**	**11**	40	**790**	<1.5
Country Fried Steak Sandwich	4	610	**33**	**12**	45	**1290**	<1.5
French Fries, regular*	4	250	**15**	**11**	5	460	<1.5
Old-Time Star Hamburger	4	450	**20**	**7**	60	**625**	<1.5
Charbroiler Steak Sandwich	4	630	**33**	—	85	**700**	<1.5
Famous Star Hamburger	4	530	**32**	**13**	70	**705**	<1.5
California Omelette	4	310	**24**	—	**630**	550	<1.5
English Muffin with Butter & Jelly*†	3	228	**9**	—	25	245	<1.5
Sweet Roll with Butter*†	3	420	**18**	—	20	450	<1.5
Taco Salad-to-Go	3	356	**19**	**6**	99	690	<1.5
Boston Clam Chowder*	3	140	**8**	**3**	22	**861**	<1.5
Sunrise Sandwich with Bacon	3	410	**24**	**8**	**310**	780	<1.5
Western Bacon Cheeseburger	3	670	**40**	**15**	90	**1330**	<1.5
Double Western Bacon Cheeseburger	3	890	**53**	**25**	**145**	**1620**	<1.5
Sausage, 1 patty*	3	110	**9**	—	25	235	<1.5
Hashed Brown Potatoes*	3	280	**19**	**4**	15	260	<1.5
Chocolate Cake*†	3	380	**20**	**6**	70	335	<1.5
Bacon, 2 strips*	3	70	**6**	**3**	10	220	<1.5
Bacon 'n Cheese Omelet	3	290	**28**	—	**470**	660	<1.5
Chocolate Chip Cookie*†	2	353	**16**	**7**	15	202	<1.5
Carrot Cake*†	2	350	**18**	—	45	375	<1.5
Sunrise Sandwich with Sausage*	2	450	**27**	**12**	**125**	790	<1.5
Scrambled Eggs	2	150	**12**	**4**	**380**	110	<1.5

* LOSES ADDITIONAL POINTS DUE TO LOW VITAMIN AND MINERAL CONTENT.

† LOSES ADDITIONAL POINT DUE TO HIGH SUGAR.

NOTE: BOLDFACE NUMBERS INDICATE NUTRITIONAL FACTOR THAT DETRACTS FROM FOOD'S NUTRITIONAL VALUE (see the note on page 22).

DAIRY QUEEN

	Rating	Calories	Fat (g)	Saturated Fat (g)	Cholesterol (mg)	Sodium (mg)	Fiber (g)
Chocolate Malt, regular*	7	760	18	—	50	260	<1.5
Parfait*	6	430	8	—	30	140	<1.5
Banana Split*	6	540	11	—	30	150	<1.5
Strawberry Shortcake*	6	540	11	—	25	215	<1.5
Soft Ice Cream Cone, regular*†	5	240	7	—	15	80	<1.5
Chocolate Sundae, regular*†	5	310	8	—	20	120	<1.5

DAIRY QUEEN (continued)

	Rating	Calories	Fat (g)	Saturated Fat (g)	Cholesterol (mg)	Sodium (mg)	Fiber (g)
Single Hamburger with Cheese	5	410	**20**	—	50	**790**	<1.5
DQ Sandwich*†	4	140	4	—	5	40	<1.5
Soft Ice Cream (without cone)*†	4	180	**6**	4	15	65	<1.5
French Fries, regular†	4	200	**10**	—	10	115	<1.5
Onion Rings†	4	280	**16**	—	15	140	<1.5
Double Hamburger	4	530	**28**	—	85	**660**	<1.5
Single Hamburger†	3	360	**16**	—	45	**630**	<1.5
Double Delight*†	3	490	**20**	—	25	150	<1.5
Hot Fudge Brownie Delight*†	3	600	**25**	—	20	225	<1.5
Chicken Sandwich†	3	670	**41**	—	75	**870**	<1.5
Double Hamburger with Cheese	3	650	**37**	—	**95**	**980**	<1.5
Dipped Chocolate Cone, regular*†	3	340	**16**	—	20	100	<1.5
Triple Hamburger	3	710	**45**	—	**135**	**690**	<1.5
Triple Hamburger with Cheese	3	820	**50**	—	**145**	**1010**	<1.5
Fish Sandwich, fried†	3	400	**17**	—	50	**875**	<1.5
Hot Dog with Cheese†	3	330	**21**	—	55	**990**	<1.5
Super Hot Dog†	3	520	**27**	—	80	**1365**	<1.5
Hot Dog†	2	280	**16**	—	45	**830**	<1.5
Dilly Bar*†	2	210	**13**	—	10	50	<1.5
Super Hot Dog with Chili†	2	570	**32**	—	**100**	**1595**	<1.5
Super Hot Dog with Cheese†	2	580	**34**	—	**100**	**1605**	<1.5
Buster Bar*†	2	460	**29**	—	10	175	<1.5
Hot Dog with Chili†	2	320	**20**	—	55	**985**	<1.5
Fish Sandwich with Cheese†	2	440	**21**	—	60	**1035**	<1.5

* LOSES ADDITIONAL POINT DUE TO HIGH SUGAR CONTENT.

† LOSES ADDITIONAL POINTS DUE TO LOW VITAMIN AND MINERAL CONTENT.

NOTE: BOLDFACE NUMBERS INDICATE NUTRITIONAL FACTOR THAT DETRACTS FROM FOOD'S NUTRITIONAL VALUE (see the note on page 22).

DOMINO'S

	Rating	Calories	Fat (g)	Saturated Fat (g)	Cholesterol (mg)	Sodium (mg)	Fiber (g)
2 Slices (Large—16") Cheese	9	376	10	**5.5**	19	483	6.4
2 Slices Ham	8	417	11	**6**	26	**805**	2.1
2 Slices Sausage/Mushroom	7	430	**15.8**	**7.7**	28	552	7.6
2 Slices Veggie (mushrooms, onion, green pepper, double cheese, & olives)	6	498	**18.5**	**10**	36	**1035**	8

DOMINO'S (continued)

	Rating	Calories	Fat (g)	Saturated Fat (g)	Cholesterol (mg)	Sodium (mg)	Fiber (g)
2 Slices Pepperoni	6	460	**17.5**	**8.4**	28	**825**	4.5
2 Slices Deluxe (sausage, pepperoni, onion, green pepper, & mushrooms)	5	498	**20.4**	**9.3**	40	**954**	7
2 Slices Double Cheese/Pepperoni	5	545	**25.3**	**13.3**	48	**1042**	8

NOTE: BOLDFACE NUMBERS INDICATE NUTRITIONAL FACTOR THAT DETRACTS FROM FOOD'S NUTRITIONAL VALUE (see the note on page 22).

HARDEE'S

	Rating	Calories	Fat (g)	Saturated Fat (g)	Cholesterol (mg)	Sodium (mg)	Fiber (g)
Chicken 'n' Pasta Salad w/1 tbsp. low-cal dressing	10	239	4	1	55	507	>1.5
Side Salad w/1 tbsp. low-cal dressing	9	29	1	trace	0	142	>1.5
Grilled Chicken Sandwich (includes lettuce & tomato)	9	310	9	1	60	**890**	>1.5
Chicken Fillet Sandwich	7	370	**13**	2	55	**1060**	<1.5
Turkey Club Sandwich (includes lettuce, tomato, & bacon)*	6	390	**16**	4	70	**1280**	>1.5
Three Pancakes w/Syrup and Margarine/Butter Blend*†	6	405	6	1	20	**955**	<1.5
Hamburger*	6	270	**10**	**4**	20	490	<1.5
Hot Ham 'n' Cheese Sandwich	6	330	**12**	**5**	65	**1420**	<1.5
Three Pancakes w/2 Bacon Strips, Syrup and Margarine/Butter Blend*†	6	505	13	3	30	**1175**	<1.5
Cool Twist Sundae (Caramel)*†	6	330	10	**5**	20	290	<1.5
Cool Twist Sundae (Strawberry)*†	5	260	8	**5**	15	115	<1.5
French Fries, regular*	5	230	**11**	2	0	85	<1.5
Rise 'n' Shine Biscuit*	5	320	**18**	3	0	**740**	<1.5
Garden Salad w/1 tbsp. low-cal dressing	5	219	**15**	**8**	105	397	>1.5
Regular Roast Beef Sandwich*	5	260	**9**	**4**	35	**730**	<1.5
9-Piece Chicken Stix*	5	310	**14**	3	55	**1020**	<1.5
Fisherman's Fillet Sandwich	5	500	**24**	6	70	**1030**	<1.5
Chicken Biscuit	5	430	**22**	4	45	**1330**	<1.5
Three Pancakes w/1 Sausage Pattie, Syrup and Margarine/Butter Blend*†	5	585	**20**	6	45	**1355**	<1.5
Country Ham Biscuit*	5	350	**18**	3	25	**1550**	<1.5
Cool Twist Cone (Chocolate or Vanilla/Chocolate)*†	5	190–200	6	**4**	20	65–80	<1.5
6-Piece Chicken Stix*	4	210	**9**	2	35	**680**	<1.5
Hash Rounds*	4	230	**14**	**3**	0	560	<1.5
Chef Salad w/1 tbsp. low-cal dressing	4	284	**16**	9	115	**1057**	>1.5
Crispy Curls*	4	300	**16**	3	0	**840**	<1.5

HARDEE'S (continued)

	Rating	Calories	Fat (g)	Saturated Fat (g)	Cholesterol (mg)	Sodium (mg)	Fiber (g)
Cinnamon 'n' Raisin*†	4	320	**17**	**5**	0	510	<1.5
Steak Biscuit*	4	500	**29**	**7**	30	**1320**	<1.5
Cool Twist Cone (Vanilla)*†	4	190	6	**4**	15	100	<1.5
Cheeseburger	4	320	**14**	**7**	30	**710**	<1.5
Cool Twist Sundae (Hot Fudge)*†	4	320	**12**	**6**	25	270	<1.5
Bacon Biscuit*	4	360	**21**	**4**	10	**950**	<1.5
Mushroom 'n' Swiss Burger	4	490	**27**	**13**	70	**940**	<1.5
¼ lb. Cheeseburger	4	500	**29**	**14**	70	**1060**	<1.5
Big Deluxe Burger	4	500	**30**	**12**	70	**760**	<1.5
Steak & Egg Biscuit	4	550	**32**	**8**	175	**1370**	<1.5
Bacon Cheeseburger	4	610	**39**	**16**	80	**1030**	<1.5
Ham & Egg Biscuit*	4	370	**19**	**4**	160	**1050**	<1.5
Ham, Egg, & Cheese Biscuit	4	420	**23**	**6**	170	**1270**	<1.5
Big Country Breakfast (Ham)	4	620	**33**	**7**	325	**1780**	<1.5
Country Ham & Egg Biscuit*	4	400	**22**	**4**	175	**1600**	<1.5
Big Country Breakfast (Country Ham)	4	670	**38**	**9**	345	**2870**	<1.5
Biscuit 'n' Gravy*	4	440	24	**6**	15	**1250**	<1.5
Big Country Breakfast (Bacon)	4	660	**40**	**10**	305	**1540**	<1.5
Sausage Biscuit*	4	440	**28**	**7**	25	**1100**	<1.5
Sausage & Egg Biscuit*	3	490	**31**	**8**	170	**1150**	<1.5
Apple Turnover*†	3	270	**12**	**4**	0	250	<1.5
Ham Biscuit	3	320	**16**	2	15	**1000**	<1.5
All Beef Hot Dog*	3	300	**17**	**8**	25	**710**	<1.5
Big Cookie*†	3	250	**13**	**4**	5	240	<1.5
Canadian Rise 'n' Shine Biscuit	3	470	**27**	**8**	180	**1550**	<1.5
Bacon, 3 strips, & Egg Biscuit*	3	410	**24**	**5**	155	**990**	<1.5
Bacon, Egg, & Cheese Biscuit	3	460	**28**	**8**	165	**1220**	<1.5
Big Country Breakfast (Sausage)	3	850	**57**	**16**	340	**1980**	<1.5

* LOSES ADDITIONAL POINTS DUE TO LOW VITAMIN AND MINERAL CONTENT.

† LOSES ADDITIONAL POINTS DUE TO HIGH SUGAR CONTENT.

NOTE: BOLDFACE NUMBERS INDICATE NUTRITIONAL FACTOR THAT DETRACTS FROM FOOD'S NUTRITIONAL VALUE (see the note on page 22).

JACK IN THE BOX

	Rating	Calories	Fat (g)	Saturated Fat (g)	Cholesterol (mg)	Sodium (mg)	Fiber (g)
Chicken Fajita Pita (includes lettuce, tomato, onions, & cheese)	9	292	8	2.9	34	**703**	>1.5
Club Pita without sauce*	7	277	8	**3.6**	43	**931**	>1.5
Beef Fajita Pita	5	333	**14**	**5.9**	45	**635**	>1.5
Mexican Chicken Salad	5	443	**21**	**7.3**	104	**1530**	>1.5
Hamburger*	5	267	**11**	**4.1**	26	556	<1.5
6-Piece Chicken Strips	4	523	**20**	**10**	103	**1122**	<1.5
Hot Club Supreme	4	524	**28**	**9.4**	82	**1467**	<1.5
Cheeseburger	4	315	**14**	**5.7**	41	**746**	<1.5
5-Piece Egg Rolls	4	675	**32**	**12**	50	**1505**	<1.5
Chef Salad w/1 tbsp. low-cal French dressing	4	345	**19**	**8.6**	142	**975**	>1.5
Taco*	4	191	**11**	**5.2**	21	406	<1.5
Taco Salad	4	641	**38**	**15.5**	91	**1670**	>1.5
Onion rings*	4	382	**23**	**11.1**	27	407	<1.5
Bacon Cheeseburger	4	705	**39**	**15**	85	**1127**	<1.5
Double Cheeseburger	4	467	**27**	**12.3**	72	**842**	<1.5
Fish Supreme	4	554	**32**	**13.5**	66	**1047**	<1.5
10-Piece Shrimp	4	270	**16**	**7.2**	84	**669**	<1.5
Side Salad w/1 tbsp. low-cal French dressing*	4	71	**4**	**2.2**	<1	159	>1.5
Breakfast Jack	3	307	**13**	**5.2**	203	**871**	<1.5
3-Piece Egg Rolls*	3	405	**19**	**7.2**	30	**903**	<1.5
Pancake Platter*	3	612	**22**	**8.6**	99	**888**	<1.5
French Fries, regular*	3	221	**12**	**5**	8	164	<1.5
Super Taco*	3	288	**17**	**8**	37	**765**	<1.5
15-Piece Shrimp	3	404	**24**	**10.8**	126	**1003**	<1.5
Scrambled Egg Platter	3	662	**40**	**17.1**	354	**1188**	<1.5
Hash Browns*	3	116	**7**	**3.6**	3	211	<1.5
Chicken Supreme*	3	575	**36**	**14.3**	62	**1525**	<1.5
Jumbo Jack with Cheese	3	677	**40**	**14**	102	**1090**	<1.5
Canadian Crescent	3	452	**31**	**9.7**	226	**851**	<1.5
Supreme Crescent	3	547	**40**	**13.2**	178	**1053**	<1.5
Sausage Crescent	3	584	**43**	**15.5**	187	**1012**	<1.5
Ultimate Cheeseburger	3	942	**69**	**26.4**	127	**1176**	<1.5
4-Piece Chicken Strips*	3	349	**14**	**6.8**	68	**748**	<1.5
Jumbo Jack*	3	584	**34**	**11**	73	**733**	<1.5
Cheesecake*†	2	309	**17.5**	**9**	63	208	<1.5
Swiss and Bacon Burger*	2	678	**47**	**20**	92	**1458**	<1.5
Hot Apple Turnover*	2	410	**24**	**10.8**	15	350	<1.5

* LOSES ADDITIONAL POINTS DUE TO LOW VITAMIN AND MINERAL CONTENT.

† LOSES ADDITIONAL POINT DUE TO HIGH SUGAR CONTENT.

NOTE: BOLDFACE NUMBERS INDICATE NUTRITIONAL FACTOR THAT DETRACTS FROM FOOD'S NUTRITIONAL VALUE (SEE THE NOTE ON PAGE 22).

KENTUCKY FRIED CHICKEN

	Rating	Calories	Fat (g)	Saturated Fat (g)	Cholesterol (mg)	Sodium (mg)	Fiber (g)
Corn-on-the-cob*	8	176	3	0.5	<1	<21	1.5
Coleslaw	8	119	**6.6**	1	5	197	1.5
Mashed Potatoes & Gravy*	7	71	1.6	0.5	<1	342	<1.5
French Fries, regular*	6	244	**12**	2.6	2	139	<1.5
1 Buttermilk Biscuit*	5	232	**12**	**2.9**	1	539	<1.5
1 Original Recipe Drumstick*	4	146	**8.5**	**2.2**	67	275	<1.5
"Chicken Littles" Sandwich*	4	169	**10**	**2**	18	331	<1.5
1 Extra Crispy Drumstick*	4	173	**11**	**2.8**	65	346	<1.5
1 Original Recipe Wing*	3	178	**12**	**3**	64	372	<1.5
1 Extra Crispy Wing*	3	218	**15.6**	**4**	63	437	<1.5
1 Original Recipe Side Breast*	3	267	**16.5**	**4.2**	77	**735**	<1.5
6 Kentucky Nuggets*	3	276	**17**	**4.2**	71	**840**	<1.5
1 Original Recipe Center Breast*	2	283	**15.3**	**3.8**	93	**672**	<1.5
1 Extra Crispy Side Breast*	2	354	**24**	**6**	66	**797**	<1.5
1 Extra Crispy Center Breast*	2	353	**21**	**5.3**	93	**842**	<1.5
1 Original Recipe Thigh*	1	294	**19.7**	**5.3**	123	**619**	<1.5
1 Extra Crispy Thigh*	1	371	**26.3**	**6.9**	121	**766**	<1.5

* LOSES ADDITIONAL POINTS DUE TO LOW VITAMIN AND MINERAL CONTENT.

NOTE: BOLDFACE NUMBERS INDICATE NUTRITIONAL FACTOR THAT DETRACTS FROM FOOD'S NUTRITIONAL VALUE (see the note on page 22).

LONG JOHN SILVER'S

	Rating	Calories	Fat (g)	Saturated Fat (g)	Cholesterol (mg)	Sodium (mg)	Fiber (g)
1 order Mixed Vegetables	9	60	2	0.6	0	330	**<1.5**
1 scoop Seafood Salad*	8	210	5	0.8	**90**	570	>1.5
1 ear Corn-on-the-Cob with Whirl	8	270	**14**	2.6	<5	95	>1.5
Seafood Salad (5 oz. lettuce mix, 5 oz. seafood salad, 2 tomato wedges, & 2 club crackers)	8	270	7	0.8	**90**	670	>1.5
Ocean Chef Salad (5 oz. lettuce mix, 2 oz. salad shrimp, 2 oz. surimi crab, ¾ oz. cheese, ½ oz. carrots, 1 tomato wedge, & 2 club crackers) w/ 1 tbsp. low-cal dressing	8	259	**9.5**	0.9	80	**1675**	>1.5
Side Salad (lettuce mix, carrots, & tomato wedge) w/1 tbsp. low-cal dressing	7	29	>.5	0.2	<3	355	**<1.5**

LONG JOHN SILVER'S (continued)

	Rating	Calories	Fat (g)	Saturated Fat (g)	Cholesterol (mg)	Sodium (mg)	Fiber (g)
Garden Salad (5 oz. lettuce mix, 1 oz. cheese, & 3 tomato wedges)	7	149	8.5	<5	<5	635	>1.5
1 Hushpuppy*	7	70	2	0.4	<5	25	<1.5
Homestyle Fish Sandwich Platter (Fish sandwich, Fryes, & Slaw)	7	870	38	8.4	55	1110	>1.5
Clam Chowder with Cod*	6	140	6	1.8	20	590	<1.5
1 order Coleslaw*	6	140	6	1	15	260	>1.5
1 piece Homestyle Fish	6	125	7	1.6	20	200	<1.5
1 piece Catfish Filet	6	180	11	2.6	25	300	<1.5
Crispy Breaded Fish Sandwich	6	600	28	6.3	30	1220	<1.5
Shrimp & Fish Dinner (1 Fish, 3 Battered Shrimp, Fryes, Slaw, & 2 Hushpuppies)*	6	770	37	8.3	80	1250	>1.5
Fish & More (2 Fish, Fryes, Slaw & 2 Hushpuppies)*	6	800	37	8.3	70	1390	>1.5
3-piece Chicken Plank Dinner (3 Chicken Planks, Fryes, Slaw, & 2 Hushpuppies)*	6	830	39	9	55	1340	>1.5
Shrimp, Fish, & Chicken Dinner (2 Battered Shrimp, 1 Fish, 1 Chicken Plank, Fryes, Slaw & 2 Hushpuppies)*	6	840	40	9	80	1450	>1.5
Breaded Shrimp Feast (13 piece Breaded Shrimp, Fryes, Slaw, & 2 Hushpuppies)	6	880	41	9	90	1320	>1.5
Catfish Fillet Dinner (2 Catfish Fillets, Fryes, Slaw, & 2 Hushpuppies)	6	860	42	9.7	65	990	>1.5
3-piece Homestyle Fish Dinner (3 Homestyle Fish, Fryes, Slaw, & 2 Hushpuppies)	6	880	42	9.5	75	980	>1.5
4-Piece Chicken Plank Dinner*	6	940	44	10.3	70	1660	>1.5
Clam Dinner (Clams, Fryes, Slaw, & 2 Hushpuppies)*	6	980	45	10	15	1200	>1.5
Seafood Platter (1 Fish, 2 Battered Shrimp, Clams, Fryes, Slaw, & 2 Hushpuppies)*	6	970	46	10.3	70	1540	>1.5
1 slice Lemon Meringue Pie*†	6	260	7	2.5	<5	270	<1.5
1 order Breaded Shrimp*	5	190	10	2.3	40	470	<1.5
1 order Breaded Clams	5	240	12	2.6	<5	410	<1.5
2-Piece Fish & Fryes (2 Fish, & 2 Hushpuppies)*	5	660	30	7.3	60	1120	<1.5
3-Piece Fish Dinner (3 Fish, Fryes, Slaw, & 2 Hushpuppies)*	5	960	44	10	100	1890	>1.5
1 piece Chicken Plank*	4	110	6	1.4	15	320	<1.5
Gumbo with Cod and Shrimp Bobs	4	120	8	2	25	740	<1.5
1 order Fryes*	4	220	10	2.6	<5	60	<1.5
1 piece Battered Fish*	4	150	8	1.8	30	510	<1.5
1 Fish, Fryes, and 1 Hushpuppy*	4	440	20	5	30	590	<1.5
6-Piece Battered Shrimp Dinner (6 Battered Shrimp, Fryes, Slaw, & 2 Hushpuppies)*	4	740	37	8.3	90	1110	>1.5
3-Piece Fish & Fryes (3 Fish, Fryes, & 2 Hushpuppies)*	4	810	38	9	85	1630	<1.5
9-Piece Battered Shrimp Dinner*	4	860	45	10	125	1470	>1.5

LONG JOHN SILVER'S (continued)

	Rating	Calories	Fat (g)	Saturated Fat (g)	Cholesterol (mg)	Sodium (mg)	Fiber (g)
1 Slice Pecan Pie*†	4	530	**25**	**7.2**	70	470	<1.5
2 Planks, Fryes, and 1 Hushpuppy*	3	510	**24**	**6**	30	**730**	<1.5
1 Fish, 1 Plank, Fryes, and 1 Hushpuppy*	3	550	**26**	**6.3**	45	**910**	<1.5

* LOSES ADDITIONAL POINTS DUE TO LOW VITAMIN AND MINERAL CONTENT (COMPLETE MEALS HAVE TO MEET MORE OF THE USRDA THAN SINGLE ITEMS DO).
† LOSES ADDITIONAL POINT DUE TO HIGH SUGAR CONTENT.

NOTE: BOLDFACE NUMBERS INDICATE NUTRITIONAL FACTOR THAT DETRACTS FROM FOOD'S NUTRITIONAL VALUE (see the note on page 22).

MCDONALD'S

	Rating	Calories	Fat (g)	Saturated Fat (g)	Cholesterol (mg)	Sodium (mg)	Fiber (g)
Chunky Chicken Salad (iceberg lettuce, green peppers, celery, tomato & sliced carrots) w/1 tbsp. Lite Vinaigrette Dressing	10	140	3.4	0.9	78	230	>1.5
Strawberry Low-fat Frozen Yogurt Sundae*	8	210	1.1	0.6	5	95	<1.5
Apple Bran Muffin*†	7	190	0	0	0	230	>1.5
English Muffin with Butter†	7	170	4.6	**2.4**	9	270	<1.5
Hot Caramel Low-fat Frozen Yogurt Sundae*†	7	270	2.8	1.5	13	180	<1.5
Hot Fudge Low-fat Frozen Yogurt Sundae*†	7	240	3.2	2.4	6	170	<1.5
McDonaldland Cookies*†	7	290	9.2	1.9	0	300	<1.5
McLean Burger	6	320	10	4	60	670	<1.5
Vanilla Cone*†	6	100	0.8	0.4	3	80	<1.5
Garden Salad (iceberg lettuce, celery, carrot, radish, cucumber, egg, tomato, & cheddar cheese) w/1 tbsp. Lite Dressing	6	125	**7.1**	**3**	83	235	>1.5
Hotcakes with Syrup & Butter*†	6	410	9.2	3.7	21	**640**	<1.5
Hamburger†	6	260	**9.5**	**3.6**	37	500	<1.5
Chef Salad (turkey, ham, cheese, egg, tomato, iceberg lettuce, celery, radish & cucumber) w/1 tbsp. Lite Dressing	5	245	**13.8**	**6**	**128**	565	>1.5
McChicken Sandwich†	5	490	**28.6**	5.4	43	**780**	<1.5
Egg McMuffin	5	290	**11.2**	**3.8**	**226**	**740**	<1.5
Apple, Raspberry, and Cinnamon Raisin Danishes*†	5	390–440	**16–21**	3.1–4.2	25–34	110–117	<1.5
Chicken McNuggets, 6 pieces†	4	270	**15.4**	**3.5**	56	580	<1.5
Cheeseburger	4	310	**13.8**	**5.2**	53	**750**	<1.5
Fillet-O-Fish†	4	440	**26.1**	**5.2**	50	**1030**	<1.5
Sausage McMuffin	4	320	**21.9**	**7.8**	64	**830**	<1.5
Quarter Pounder	4	410	**20.7**	**8.1**	86	**660**	<1.5
Fries, Medium†	3	320	**17.1**	**7.2**	12	150	<1.5
Hashbrown Potatoes†	3	130	**7.3**	**3.2**	9	330	<1.5

MCDONALD'S (continued)

	Rating	Calories	Fat (g)	Saturated Fat (g)	Cholesterol (mg)	Sodium (mg)	Fiber (g)
Biscuit, with Biscuit Spread†	3	260	**12.7**	**3.4**	1	**730**	<1.5
Scrambled Eggs†	3	140	**9.8**	**3.3**	399	290	<1.5
Apple Pie*†	3	260	**14.8**	**4.8**	0	240	<1.5
Chocolaty Chip Cookies, 1 box*†	3	330	**15.6**	**5**	4	280	<1.5
Iced Cheese Danish*†	3	390	**21.8**	**6**	47	420	<1.5
Quarter Pounder with Cheese	3	520	**29.2**	**11.2**	118	**1150**	<1.5
Sausage McMuffin with Egg	3	440	**26.8**	**9.5**	263	**980**	<1.5
McD.L.T.	3	580	**36.8**	**11.5**	109	**990**	<1.5
1.7 oz. Pork Sausage†	3	180	**16.3**	**5.9**	48	350	<1.5
Biscuit with Bacon, Egg, & Cheese	3	440	**26.4**	**8.2**	253	**1230**	<1.5
Biscuit with Sausage†	3	440	**29**	**9.3**	49	**1080**	<1.5
Big Mac	3	560	**32.4**	**10.1**	103	**950**	<1.5
Biscuit with Sausage, Egg†	2	520	**34.5**	**11.2**	275	**1250**	<1.5

* LOSES ADDITIONAL POINT DUE TO HIGH SUGAR CONTENT.

† LOSES ADDITIONAL POINTS DUE TO LOW VITAMIN AND MINERAL CONTENT.

NOTE: BOLDFACE NUMBERS INDICATE NUTRITIONAL FACTOR THAT DETRACTS FROM FOOD'S NUTRITIONAL VALUE (see the note on page 22).

PIZZA HUT

	Rating	Calories	Fat (g)	Saturated Fat (g)	Cholesterol (mg)	Sodium (mg)	Fiber (g)
2 Slices Cheese Pan Pizza	6	492	**18**	**9**	34	**940**	5
2 Slices Cheese Hand-Tossed Pizza	6	518	**20**	**14**	55	**1276**	7
2 Slices Cheese Thin 'n Crispy Pizza	5	398	**17**	**10**	33	**867**	4
2 Slices Pepperoni Thin 'n Crispy Pizza	5	413	**20**	**11**	46	**986**	4
2 Slices Supreme Thin 'n Crispy Pizza	5	459	**22**	**11**	50	**1328**	5
2 Slices Super Supreme Thin 'n Crispy Pizza (cheese, pepperoni, sausage, mushrooms, green peppers, & olives)	5	463	**21**	**10**	56	**1336**	5
2 Slices Pepperoni Pan Pizza	5	540	**22**	**9**	42	**1127**	5
2 Slices Supreme Pan Pizza	5	589	**30**	**14**	48	**1363**	7
2 Slices Super Supreme Pan Pizza	5	563	**26**	**12**	55	**1447**	6
2 Slices Pepperoni Hand-Tossed Pizza	5	500	**23**	**13**	50	**1267**	6
2 Slices Supreme Hand-Tossed Pizza	5	540	**26**	**14**	55	**1470**	7
2 Slices Super Supreme Hand-Tossed Pizza	5	556	**25**	**13**	54	**1648**	7
1 Pepperoni Personal Pan Pizza	5	675	**29**	**12**	53	**1335**	8
1 Supreme Personal Pan Pizza	5	647	**28**	**11**	49	**1313**	9

NOTE: BOLDFACE NUMBERS INDICATE NUTRITIONAL FACTOR THAT DETRACTS FROM FOOD'S NUTRITIONAL VALUE (see the note on page 22).

ROY ROGERS

	Rating	Calories	Fat (g)	Saturated Fat (g)	Cholesterol (mg)	Sodium (mg)	Fiber (g)
Baked Potato, plain	10	211	0	0	0	trace	1.5
Baked Potato, Hot Topped with Margarine	9	274	7	<5	0	161	1.5
Coleslaw	6	110	7	>2	0	261	1.5
Baked Potato, Hot Topped, Broccoli 'n Cheese	6	376	18	>7	0	523	1.5
Roast Beef Sandwich	6	317	10	<6	55	785	<1.5
Baked Potato, Hot Topped, Sour Cream 'n Chives	6	408	21	>7	31	138	>1.5
Baked Potato, Hot Topped, Taco Beef 'n Cheese	5	463	22	>8	37	726	>1.5
Roast Beef Sandwich, large	5	360	12	<7	73	1044	<1.5
Caramel Sundae*†	5	293	8	>5	23	193	<1.5
Hot Fudge Sundae†	5	337	13	>6	23	186	<1.5
Chicken Leg*	4	117	7	<2	64	162	<1.5
Chicken Wing*	4	142	10	<3	52	266	<1.5
French Fries, regular*	4	268	14	>5	42	165	<1.5
Pancake Platter, with Syrup & Butter*†	4	452	15	>7	53	842	<1.5
Pancake Platter with Ham, Syrup, & Butter†	4	506	17	>8	73	1264	<1.5
Pancake Platter with Bacon, Syrup, & Butter†	4	493	18	>8	63	1065	<1.5
Roast Beef Sandwich with Cheese*	4	424	19	>7	77	1694	<1.5
Chicken Thigh*	4	282	20	>4	89	505	<1.5
Baked Potato, Hot Topped, Bacon 'n' Cheese*	4	397	22	>7	34	778	1.5
Hamburger Sandwich*	4	456	28	>8	73	495	<1.5
Strawberry Sundae*†	4	216	7	>3	23	99	<1.5
Roast Beef with Cheese, large	3	467	21	>8	95	1953	<1.5
Biscuit*	3	231	12	>4	0	575	<1.5
Cheeseburger	3	563	37	>9	95	1404	<1.5
Strawberry Shortcake†	3	447	19	>8	28	674	<1.5
RR Bar Burger	3	611	39	>11	115	1826	<1.5
Crescent Roll*	3	287	18	>5	0	547	<1.5
Bacon Cheeseburger	3	581	39	>10	103	1536	<1.5
Breakfast Crescent Sandwich with Ham	3	557	42	>10	189	1192	<1.5
Potato Salad*	2	107	6	>2	0	696	<1.5
Macaroni*	2	186	11	>3	0	603	<1.5
Chicken Breast*	2	324	19	<6	324	601	<1.5
Chicken Thigh & Leg*	2	399	26	<6	153	667	<1.5
Chicken Breast & Wing*	2	466	29	<9	376	867	<1.5
Brownie*†	2	264	11	>4	10	150	<1.5
Cheese Danish*†	2	254	12	>4	11	260	<1.5
Cherry Danish*†	2	271	14	>4	11	242	<1.5
Apple Danish*†	2	249	12	>4	15	255	<1.5
Breakfast Crescent Sandwich*	2	401	27	>7	148	867	<1.5
Egg & Biscuit Platter*	2	394	27	>7	284	734	<1.5

ROY ROGERS (continued)

	Rating	Calories	Fat (g)	Saturated Fat (g)	Cholesterol (mg)	Sodium (mg)	Fiber (g)
Pancake Platter with Sausage, Syrup, & Butter*	2	608	30	>10	94	1167	<1.5
Breakfast Crescent Sandwich with Sausage*	2	449	29	>7	168	1289	<1.5
Breakfast Crescent Sandwich with Bacon*	2	431	30	>7	156	1035	<1.5
Egg & Biscuit Platter with Ham*	2	442	29	>7	304	1156	<1.5
Egg & Biscuit Platter with Bacon*	2	435	30	>7	294	957	<1.5
Egg & Biscuit Platter with Sausage*	2	550	41	>9	325	1059	<1.5

* LOSES ADDITIONAL POINTS DUE TO LOW VITAMIN AND MINERAL CONTENT.

† LOSES ADDITIONAL POINT DUE TO HIGH SUGAR CONTENT.

NOTE: BOLDFACE NUMBERS INDICATE NUTRITIONAL FACTOR THAT DETRACTS FROM FOOD'S NUTRITIONAL VALUE (see the note on page 22).

Note: Hardee's recently purchased Roy Rogers and some menu changes may occur as a result.

TACO BELL

	Rating	Calories	Fat (g)	Saturated Fat (g)	Cholesterol (mg)	Sodium (mg)	Fiber (g)
Bean Burrito with green or red sauce	9	351–357	10	3	9	**763–888**	>1.5
Tostada with green or red sauce	6	237–243	**11**	**4**	16	471–596	>1.5
Pintos & Cheese with green sauce	6	184	**8**	**4**	16	518	>1.5
Super Combo Taco	6	286	**16**	**7**	40	462	>1.5
Soft Taco Supreme	6	275	**16**	**8**	32	516	>1.5
Taco BellGrande	6	355	**23**	**11**	56	472	>1.5
Burrito Supreme with green or red sauce	5	407–413	**18**	**8**	33	**796–921**	>1.5
Pintos & Cheese with red sauce	5	190	**9**	**4**	16	**642**	>1.5
Chicken Fajita	5	226	**10**	**4**	44	**619**	<1.5
Double Beef Burrito Supreme with green or red sauce	5	451–457	**22**	**10**	57	**928–1053**	>1.5
Steak Fajita	5	234	**11**	**5**	14	485	<1.5
Nachos	5	346	**18**	**6**	9	399	<1.5
Nachos BellGrande	5	649	**35**	**12**	36	**997**	>1.5
Taco Salad with salsa without shell	5	520	**31**	**14**	80	**1431**	>1.5
Taco Salad with salsa & shell	5	941	**61**	**19**	80	**1662**	>1.5
Mexican Pizza	5	575	**37**	**11**	52	**1031**	>1.5
Taco Light	5	410	**29**	**12**	56	594	<1.5
Enchirito with green or red sauce	4	371–382	**20**	**9**	54	**993–1243**	<1.5
Beef Burrito with green or red sauce	4	398–403	**17**	**7**	57	**926–1051**	<1.5
Soft Taco*	4	228	**12**	**5**	32	516	<1.5
Taco*	4	183	**11**	**5**	32	276	<1.5

TACO BELL (continued)

	Rating	Calories	Fat (g)	Saturated Fat (g)	Cholesterol (mg)	Sodium (mg)	Fiber (g)
Meximelt	4	266	15	8	38	**689**	<1.5
Cinnamon Crispas†	4	259	15	4	1	127	<1.5

* LOSES ADDITIONAL POINTS DUE TO LOW VITAMIN AND MINERAL CONTENT.

† LOSES ADDITIONAL POINT DUE TO HIGH SUGAR CONTENT.

NOTE: BOLDFACE NUMBERS INDICATE NUTRITIONAL FACTOR THAT DETRACTS FROM FOOD'S NUTRITIONAL VALUE (see the note on page 22).

WENDY'S

	Rating	Calories	Fat (g)	Saturated Fat (g)	Cholesterol (mg)	Sodium (mg)	Fiber (g)
Baked Potato, plain	10	270	<1	trace	0	20	>1.5
Baked Potato with Cheese	9	420	**15**	4	10	310	>1.5
Garden Salad (lettuce, tomatoes, cauliflower, broccoli, imitation cheese, & cucumbers) w/1 tbsp. low-cal dressing	8	127	**7**	N/A	0	295	>1.5
Chili, 9 oz.	8	220	7	**2.6**	45	**750**	>1.5
Baked Potato with Broccoli & Cheese	8	400	**16**	2.9	trace	455	>1.5
Baked Potato with Bacon & Cheese	8	520	**18**	5.1	20	**1460**	>1.5
Chef Salad (lettuce, tomatoes, eggs, cauliflower, carrots, broccoli, imitation cheese, turkey-ham, white turkey, & cucumbers) w/1 tbsp. low-cal Italian dressing	7	205	**11**	N/A	**120**	325	>1.5
Grilled Chicken Sandwich	7	340	**13**	2.5	60	**815**	<1.5
Baked Potato with Chili & Cheese	7	500	**18**	4	25	**630**	>1.5
Frosty Dairy Dessert, small, 12 fl. oz.*	6	400	14	**4.8**	50	220	<1.5
Chicken Sandwich	6	430	**19**	2.8	60	**725**	<1.5
Baked Potoato with Sour Cream & Chives	6	500	**23**	**9.3**	25	135	>1.5
Jr. Hamburger†	6	260	**9**	**3.3**	34	570	<1.5
Kids' Meal Hamburger†	6	260	**9**	3.3	35	570	<1.5
Jr. Swiss Deluxe (2 oz. patty, swiss cheese, mayonnaise, ketchup, pickles, onion, tomato, lettuce, mustard, & bun)	6	360	**18**	3.3	40	**765**	<1.5
Chicken Club Sandwich	6	506	**25**	5	70	**930**	<1.5
Taco Salad (lettuce, chili, cheese, tomatoes, & taco chips) w/1 tbsp. low-cal bacon & tomato dressing	5	705	**41**	N/A	35	**1300**	>1.5
Plain Single Hamburger	5	340	15	**5.7**	65	500	<1.5
Jr. Cheeseburger†	5	310	13	3.2	34	**770**	<1.5
Kids' Meal Cheeseburger†	5	300	13	3.3	35	**770**	<1.5
Single with everything	5	420	**21**	**5.7**	70	**890**	<1.5
French Fries, large†	5	312	**15.6**	3.3	0	189	<1.5
Fish Fillet Sandwich†	5	460	**25**	5	55	**780**	<1.5

WENDY'S (continued)

	Rating	Calories	Fat (g)	Saturated Fat (g)	Cholesterol (mg)	Sodium (mg)	Fiber (g)
Jr. Bacon Cheeseburger	5	430	**25**	**5.5**	50	**835**	**<1.5**
Big Classic (¼ lb. beef patty, mayonnaise, ketchup, pickles, onions, tomatoes, lettuce, & bun)	5	570	**33**	5.9	**90**	**1085**	**<1.5**
Plain Single Cheeseburger	4	410	**21**	**9.2**	80	**760**	**<1.5**
Big Classic with Cheese	4	640	**39**	**9.4**	105	**1345**	**<1.5**
Breakfast Sandwich (white bread, egg, & cheese)	3	370	**19**	N/A	**200**	**770**	**<1.5**
Home Fries*	3	360	**22**	N/A	20	**745**	**<1.5**
Scrambled Eggs†	3	190	**12**	N/A	**450**	160	**<1.5**
Sausage, 1 patty†	3	200	**18**	N/A	30	410	**<1.5**
Crispy Chicken Nuggets (6)†	3	280	**20**	4.5	50	**600**	**<1.5**
Chocolate Chip Cookie*†	3	275	**13**	**4.2**	15	256	**<1.5**
Bacon, 2 strips†	2	110	**10**	N/A	15	445	**<1.5**
Danish*†	1	360	**18**	N/A	N/A	340	**<1.5**

* LOSES ADDITIONAL POINTS DUE TO LOW VITAMIN AND MINERAL CONTENT.

† LOSES ADDITIONAL POINT DUE TO HIGH SUGAR CONTENT.

NOTE: BOLDFACE NUMBERS INDICATE NUTRITIONAL FACTOR THAT DETRACTS FROM FOOD'S NUTRITIONAL VALUE (see the note on page 22).

BOXED MEALS

	Rating	Calories	Fat (g)	Saturated Fat (g)	Cholesterol (mg)	Sodium (mg)	Fiber (g)
¼ Thin Crust Cheese Pizza from Contadina Pizzeria Kit	9	209	3	0.2	0	**650**	>1.5
¼ Thick Crust Cheese Pizza from Contadina Pizzeria Kit	9	295	3.8	0.2	0	**820**	>1.5
4 oz. Hunt's Minute Gourmet with 3.7 oz. chicken*	8	300	4	<3	<90	420	<1.5
¾ c. Kraft Macaroni & Cheese Deluxe Dinner, unsalted cooking water*	7	260	8	**4**	20	590	<1.5
⅙ package Betty Crocker Suddenly Salad, average of Classic Pasta & Italian Pasta	6	155	**7**	<4	<90	340	>1.5
¾ c. Kraft Macaroni & Cheese with whole milk, margarine, & no salt added*	7	290	**13**	3	5	530	<1.5
¾ c. Velveeta Pasta Shells & Cheese, no salt added*	4	260	**10**	5	25	**720**	<1.5
⅕ package Tuna Helper Main Dishes with 1.3 oz. tuna, average of 6 varieties*	4	300	**13.8**	<4	<90	**943**	<1.5
1 burger made with Oscar Mayer Onion Burger Stuffing*	4	229	**16.9**	>6	88	452	<1.5
1 burger made with Oscar Mayer Mushroom Burger Stuffing*	4	224	**17.3**	>6	65	440	<1.5

BOXED MEALS (continued)

	Rating	Calories	Fat (g)	Saturated Fat (g)	Cholesterol (mg)	Sodium (mg)	Fiber (g)
1 burger made with Oscar Mayer Bacon & Cheese Burger Stuffing*	4	265	19.8	>6	71	588	<1.5
⅕ package Chicken Helper Main Dishes with chicken, etc. added, average for 5 varieties	4	530	27.8	<9	<90	**1116**	<1.5
⅕ package Hamburger Helper Main Dishes with ⅕ lb. ground beef added, average for 15 varieties*	3	335	15	>6	<90	**1027**	<1.5
1 burger made with Oscar Mayer Pizza Burger Stuffing*	3	244	18	>6	62	**615**	<1.5
1 burger made with Oscar Mayer Mexican Style Burger Stuffing*	3	233	18.4	>6	53	**701**	<1.5

* LOSES ADDITIONAL POINTS DUE TO LOW VITAMIN AND MINERAL CONTENTS.
NOTE: BOLDFACE NUMBERS INDICATE NUTRITIONAL FACTOR THAT DETRACTS FROM FOOD'S NUTRITIONAL VALUE (see the note on page 22).

BOXED BREADS AND RICE

	Rating	Calories	Fat (g)	Saturated Fat (g)	Cholesterol (mg)	Sodium (mg)	Fiber (g)
1 Duncan Hines bran & honey muffin from mix	7	98	2.8	<2	0	161	>1.5
½ c. Heinz Near East Rice (Chicken Flavored, Long Grain and Wild Rice Pilaf)*	7	100	0	0	0	370–400	<1.5
½ c. Heinz Near East Spanish Rice*	7	110	0	0	0	470	<1.5
1 generic piece corn bread from mix	7	178	5.8	1.7	<10	263	<1.5
1 Duncan Hines blueberry muffin from mix	6	99	2.7	<2	0	147	<1.5
1 generic corn muffin from mix	6	130	4.2	1.2	<10	192	<1.5
1 piece Cinch corn bread from mix	6	210	5	**<2**	<10	**610**	<1.5
1 Krusteaz oat bran muffin from mix	6	210	6	<4	<10	340	>1.5
1 piece Pillsbury banana bread from mix	6	170	**6**	<3	<10	200	<1.5
1 slice generic fruit quick bread from mix	5	118	2.4	<2	<10	<600	<1.5
1 generic blueberry muffin from mix	5	126	**4.3**	<2	<20	200	<1.5
1 generic biscuit from mix	5	93	**3.3**	<2	<10	262	<1.5
1 Betty Crocker oat bran muffin from mix	4	190	**8**	<4	<10	240	>1.5

* LOSE ADDITIONAL POINTS DUE TO LOW VITAMIN AND MINERAL CONTENT.
NOTE: BOLDFACE NUMBERS INDICATE NUTRITIONAL FACTOR THAT DETRACTS FROM FOOD'S NUTRITIONAL VALUE (see the note on page 22).

CANNED SOUPS

	Rating	Calories	Fat (g)	Saturated Fat (g)	Cholesterol (mg)	Sodium (mg)	Fiber (g)
1 c. Campbell's Low-Sodium Split Pea Soup	10	173	3	<2	<10	21	>1.5
1 c. Progresso Lentil Soup	9	143	1.7	<1	<10	**857**	>1.5
1 c. Campbell's Low-Sodium Tomato Soup with Tomato Pieces	9	138	3.8	<1	<10	36	**<1.5**
1 c. chunky vegetable soup	9	122	3.7	0.6	0	**1010**	>1.5
1 c. Campbell's Low-sodium Chunky Vegetable Beef Soup	9	122	3	<2	<20	51	**<1.5**
1 c. chunky split pea soup with ham	9	184	4	1.6	7	**965**	>1.5
1 c. Hain Naturals Vegetable Chicken Soup*	8	102	2.6	<1	<20	85	**<1.5**
1 c. lentil with ham soup*	8	140	2.8	1.1	7	**1318**	>1.5
1 c. Campbell's Tomato Soup	8	84	1	<1	<10	**662**	**<1.5**
1 c. Progresso Beef Vegetable Soup	8	126	1.7	<1	<20	**958**	**<1.5**
1 c. Progresso Homestyle Chicken Soup	8	76	1.7	<1	<20	**1000**	**<1.5**
1 c. Progresso Manhattan Clam Chowder	8	118	2.5	<1	<20	**1042**	**<1.5**
1 c. Progresso Chicken Noodle Soup	8	109	3.4	<2	<20	**832**	**<1.5**
1 c. Progresso Beef Minestrone Soup	8	135	3.6	<2	<20	**936**	**<1.5**
1 c. chunky chicken vegetable soup	8	167	4.8	1.4	17	**1068**	**<1.5**
1 c. Campbell's Wonton Soup	8	233	1	<1	<20	**878**	**<1.5**
1 c. chunky minestrone soup	7	127	2.8	1.5	5	**864**	**<1.5**
1 c. chunky manhattan clam chowder	7	133	3.4	**2.1**	14	**1000**	**<1.5**
1 c. Campbell's Low-Sodium Chicken Noodle Soup*	7	85	2.2	<2	<20	40	**<1.5**
1 c. Campbell's New England Clam Chowder*	7	80	2	<2	<20	**879**	**<1.5**
1 c. Progresso Chicken Vegetable Soup	7	109	**4.2**	<2	<20	**638**	**<1.5**
1 c. chunky chicken soup	7	178	**6.6**	**2**	30	**887**	**<1.5**
1 c. chunky bean with ham soup	7	231	**8.5**	**3.3**	22	**972**	>1.5
1 c. Progresso Hearty Chicken Soup	6	143	**6.7**	<3	<20	**848**	**<1.5**
1 c. Campbell's Chicken Noodle Soup*	6	60	1	<1	<20	**897**	**<1.5**
7.5 oz. Swanson Chicken & Vegetable Stew*	5	164	**7.1**	<3	<30	**962**	**<1.5**
1 c. vegetable & beef stew	5	194	**7.6**	<3	<30	**1007**	**<1.5**
1 c. Progresso French Onion Soup*	4	101	**6.7**	<5	<50	**1067**	**<1.5**
1 c. Van Camp's Chili without Beans	4	412	**33.5**	**>10**	<90	**1499**	**<1.5**

* LOSES ADDITIONAL POINTS DUE TO LOW VITAMIN AND MINERAL CONTENT.

NOTE: BOLDFACE NUMBERS INDICATE NUTRITIONAL FACTOR THAT DETRACTS FROM FOOD'S NUTRITIONAL VALUE (see the note on page 22).

OTHER CANNED GOODS

	Rating	Calories	Fat (g)	Saturated Fat (g)	Cholesterol (mg)	Sodium (mg)	Fiber (g)
1 c. baked beans with pork	9	268	3.9	1.5	17	**1048**	6.6
7.5 oz. Franco-American Beef Ravioli	8	223	4.7	<3	<60	**1092**	**<1.5**
1 c. baked beans with beef	8	321	9.2	**4.5**	59	**1264**	>1.5
7.5 oz. Franco-American Spaghettio's with Tomato & Cheese Sauce*	7	165	1.3	<1	<30	**912**	**<1.5**
7.5 oz. Franco-American Beef Raviolio's	6	293	5.3	**<4**	<60	**920**	**<1.5**
1 c. baked beans with franks	6	366	**16.9**	**6**	15	**1105**	5.9
7.4 oz. Franco-American Spaghettio's with Meatballs*	5	204	**7.5**	<3	<50	**946**	**<1.5**
7.4 oz. Franco-American Spaghettio's with Franks*	4	210	**8.4**	<3	<50	**974**	**<1.5**
1 c. macaroni & cheese*	3	228	**9.6**	**4.2**	<30	**730**	**<1.5**

* LOSES ADDITIONAL POINTS DUE TO LOW VITAMIN AND MINERAL CONTENT.

NOTE: BOLDFACE NUMBERS INDICATE NUTRITIONAL FACTOR THAT DETRACTS FROM FOOD'S NUTRITIONAL VALUE (see the note on page 22).

HOT DOGS

	Rating	Calories	Fat (g)	Saturated Fat (g)	Cholesterol (mg)	Sodium (mg)	Fiber (g)
1 turkey frank*	4	100	**8.1**	**2.7**	39	472	**0**
1 Louis Rich Turkey with Cheese Frank*	4	108	**8.6**	**3.1**	40	514	**0**
1 regular beef frank*	4	142	**12.8**	**5.4**	27	462	**0**
1 Oscar Mayer Nacho Style with Cheese Frank*	4	138	**12.5**	>3	30	550	**0**
1 Oscar Mayer Frank with Bacon & Cheddar Cheese*	4	143	**12.7**	>3	30	509	**0**
1 regular beef & pork frank*	4	144	**13.1**	**4.8**	22	504	**0**
1 Armour Low-Salt Jumbo Beef Hot Dog*	4	170	**15**	>4	27	440	**0**
1 large beef frank*	4	180	**16.5**	**6.9**	34	585	**0**
1 regular chicken frank*	3	116	**8.8**	**2.5**	45	**617**	**0**
1 Hormel Corn Dog Batter-Wrapped Wiener*	3	220	**21**	>4	<40	**656**	**<1.5**

* LOSES ADDITIONAL POINTS DUE TO LOW VITAMIN AND MINERAL CONTENT.

NOTE: ALTHOUGH CHICKEN AND TURKEY HOT DOGS PROVIDE 1½ TEASPOONS OF FAT PER OUNCE AS OPPOSED TO 2½ TEASPOONS PER OUNCE FOR BEEF HOT DOGS, THE BIGGEST VARIABLE IS IN HOW MANY OUNCES PER HOT DOG. CHOOSE THE SMALL ONES WHEN YOU HAVE A CHOICE, AND REMEMBER THAT THEIR FAT IS SATURATED FAT, ALONG WITH A SODIUM CONTENT OF 450 TO 650 MILLIGRAMS PER DOG.

NOTE: BOLD FACED NUMBERS INDICATE NUTRITIONAL FACTOR THAT DETRACTS FROM FOOD'S NUTRITIONAL VALUE (see the note on page 22).

FROZEN MEALS

	Rating	Calories	Fat (g)	Saturated Fat (g)	Cholesterol (mg)	Sodium (mg)	Fiber (g)
Healthy Choice chicken Dijon dinner	10	260	3	1	45	420	>1.5
Healthy Choice chicken enchilada dinner	10	330	6	3	25	420	>1.5
Healthy Choice pasta primavera dinner	10	280	3	2	15	360	>1.5
Healthy Choice chicken & vegetables*	9	210	<1	1	35	490	>1.5
Healthy Choice chicken fajitas*	9	200	3	1	35	310	>1.5
Healthy Choice beef fajitas*	9	210	4	2	35	250	>1.5
Healthy Choice zucchini lasagna*	9	240	3	2	15	390	>1.5
Healthy Choice chicken parmigiana dinner*	9	290	5	2	65	320	>1.5
Healthy Choice breast of turkey dinner*	9	270	5	2	55	450	>1.5
Healthy Choice chicken oriental dinner*	9	210	1	<1	45	410	>1.5
Healthy Choice sole au gratin dinner*	9	280	5	2	40	490	>1.5
Stouffer's RIGHT COURSE vegetarian chili w/seasoned rice*	9	280	7	1	0	590	>1.5
Healthy Choice chicken & pasta divan dinner*	8	310	4	2	60	560	<1.5
Healthy Choice sirloin tips dinner*	8	280	6	2	55	320	<1.5
The Budget Gourmet Light mandarin chicken*	8	290	6	<3	<90	690	>1.5
Healthy Choice lasagna w/ meat sauce*	8	250	4	2	20	420	<1.5
Light & Elegant beef teriyaki w/rice & pea pods*	8	240	3	<2	45	625	>1.5
Light & Elegant Florentine lasagna	8	280	5	<3	25	980	<1.5
Le Menu Light Style beef à l'orange*	8	290	8	<4	<60	580	<1.5
Banquet noodles & chicken	8	361	11	<5	<50	964	<1.5
Banquet turkey dinner	8	320	9	<4	<90	1416	<1.5
Le Menu LIGHT STYLE Swedish meatballs	7	260	8	3	40	700	<1.5
Banquet chicken cacciatore*	7	260	5	<3	40	510	<1.5
Light & Elegant chicken parmigiana w/parsley noodles*	7	260	6	<3	<60	680	<1.5
Light & Elegant spaghetti w/meat sauce*	7	290	8	<4	35	700	<1.5
Weight Watchers stuffed sole*	7	310	9	1	5	940	<1.5
Light & Elegant beef Stroganoff*	7	260	6	<3	65	790	>1.5
Weight Watchers spaghetti with meat sauce*	7	280	7	3	35	910	<1.5
Light & Elegant beef julienne w/rice & peppers*	7	260	7	<3	<90	990	<1.5
Healthy Choice shrimp creole dinner*	7	230	3	1	90	420	<1.5
Budget Gourmet Light sliced turkey breast w/herb gravy*	7	290	8	<4	45	1050	<1.5
Light & Elegant chicken w/broccoli*	7	290	11	<4	<60	805	>1.5
Banquet spaghetti w/meat sauce*	7	270	8	<3	<90	1242	<1.5
Banquet pasta shells & sauce*	7	310	8	<4	35	950	<1.5
Banquet fried chicken	7	359	11	<6	<90	1831	<1.5
Banquet beef enchilada*	7	497	15	<9	<90	1805	>1.5
Banquet beans & franks dinner	7	500	19	<9	34	1377	>1.5
Weight Watchers lasagna with meat sauce	7	330	11	5	60	990	>1.5

FROZEN MEALS (continued)

	Rating	Calories	Fat (g)	Saturated Fat (g)	Cholesterol (mg)	Sodium (mg)	Fiber (g)
Light & Elegant glazed chicken w/rice & vegetables*	6	240	4	<3	75	660	<1.5
Light & Elegant chicken in barbecue sauce w/corn & pecan rice*	6	300	6	<4	<90	900	<1.5
Light & Elegant beef Burgundy w/parsley noodles*	6	230	4	<3	55	1240	<1.5
Banquet chipped & creamed beef*	6	90	2	<2	25	818	<1.5
Banquet green pepper steak*	6	310	5	<4	50	1125	<1.5
Le Menu LIGHT STYLE 3-cheese stuffed shells w/broccoli*	6	280	8	>4	<90	750	1.5
Budget Gourmet Light roast chicken w/herb gravy*	6	270	9	<5	55	1010	<1.5
Budget Gourmet pepper steak w/rice*	6	300	9	<5	<90	800	<1.5
Light & Elegant mac. & cheese w/bread crumbs*	6	300	9	<5	5	1010	<1.5
Light & Elegant chicken in cheese sauce w/rice & broccoli*	6	293	11	<5	50	800	>1.5
Banquet cheese enchilada*	6	543	19	<9	<90	927	>1.5
Weight Watchers beef enchiladas ranchero	6	300	13	4	45	930	>1.5
Weight Watchers chicken enchiladas ranchero	6	360	18	5	60	900	>1.5
Stouffer's Lean Cuisine turkey Dijon	5	280	11	<5	70	1030	<1.5
Light & Elegant shrimp Creole w/rice & peppers*	5	218	2	<1	120	1050	<1.5
⅓ Totino's vegetable party pizza*	5	219	8	>4	<90	631	>1.5
Banquet lasagna with meat sauce*	5	330	11	<6	<70	1000	<1.5
1 piece Pillsbury microwave cheese French bread pizza*	5	339	13.5	>6	<90	574	>1.5
Le Menu sliced turkey breast w/mushroom gravy, rice, & vegetables	5	460	24	>8	<90	1140	>1.5
Weight Watchers oven-fried fish w/rice pilaf*	5	300	13	<1	15	500	<1.5
Banquet ham dinner	5	532	22	<9	<90	1148	<1.5
Banquet fish dinner	5	553	33	<9	<90	927	<1.5
Weight Watchers baked cheese ravioli*	4	290	12	5	85	550	<1.5
1 Weight Watchers chicken burrito w/vegetables*	4	310	13	4	60	790	<1.5
⅓ Totino's Canadian bacon party pizza*	4	230	8.4	>4	<90	670	>1.5
1 Weight Watchers beefsteak burrito w/vegetables*	4	310	13	<5	80	730	>1.5
⅓ Totino's pepperoni party pizza	4	270	13	>5	<90	772	>1.5
Le Menu chicken parmigiana dinner	4	380	18	<7	<90	890	<1.5
1 Pillsbury microwave sausage French bread pizza	4	409	19	>7	<90	1018	>1.5
1 Pillsbury microwave pepperoni French bread pizza	4	410	20	>7	<90	1163	>1.5
¼ Celeste pepperoni pizza	4	368	21	>6	<90	1061	>1.5
¼ Celeste sausage pizza	4	376	22	>6	<90	988	>1.5
Banquet beef & gravy	4	345	19	>6	<90	1009	<1.5
Banquet salisbury steak meal	4	395	26	>7	76	1333	<1.5
¼ Celeste deluxe pizza	4	378	22	>6	<90	953	>1.5
⅔ Celeste cheese pizza	4	333	16	>6	<90	555	>1.5
½ Celeste Canadian bacon pizza	4	273	13	>5	<90	797	>1.5

FROZEN MEALS (continued)

	Rating	Calories	Fat (g)	Saturated Fat (g)	Cholesterol (mg)	Sodium (mg)	Fiber (g)
Banquet meat loaf meal	4	437	27	>7	82	**1525**	**<1.5**
Banquet chopped beef meal	4	434	30	>7	76	**1199**	**<1.5**
⅓ Totino's cheese party pizza	3	255	12	>5	<90	**635**	>1.5

* LOSES POINTS DUE TO LOW VITAMIN AND MINERAL CONTENT.

NOTE: BOLDFACE NUMBERS INDICATE NUTRITIONAL FACTOR THAT DETRACTS FROM FOOD'S NUTRITIONAL VALUE (see the note on page 22).

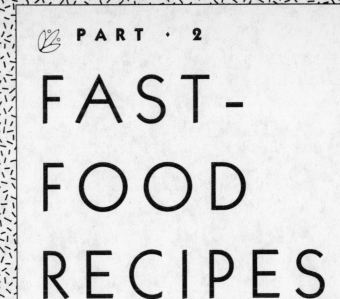

PART · 2

FAST-
FOOD
RECIPES

CHAPTER · 9

PREPARATION AND GENERAL RULES

WHY PEOPLE DON'T COOK AT HOME

You can eat Fast-Food Diet fare at home, and, quite frankly, it's your very best chance to "have it your way." With total control over food preparation, you can be sure to use the best and freshest ingredients, while adding fats in small amounts.

But for some people, cooking a meal is a rarity. Let's look at the reasons why, and determine what can be done about it.

Excuse #1: "I don't have time to cook."

Reality: Cooking healthy food doesn't have to take very much time. It just requires planning and having the foods on hand, plus the ideas to put them together tastefully and simply. That's what this part of the book is about.

Excuse #2: "It's too much trouble to cook for one person."

Reality: If you really *want* to eat healthy food at home, then you need to change your attitude. Why shouldn't you treat yourself well and prepare healthy meals for yourself? Perhaps your state of mind is task-related, and a little exercise after a long day at work will give you a new outlook, one that comes with the desire to take good care of yourself. When you are prepared to cook, a simple dish can be less trouble than getting into the car, driving, and waiting to order and be served. Besides, this gets old night after night. Think of that feeling of satisfaction you'll have after eating your own tasty, healthy food.

Excuse #3: "When I cook healthful food, the kids won't eat it."

Reality: Start children on healthful foods as young as possible. Establish ground rules for afterschool snacks, stating what kids can eat and at what times. Don't keep too many high-fat chips, baked goods, or soft drinks in the house. Make other, nutritious snacks available, such as grapes, watermelon cubes, whole wheat crackers and peanut butter, unbuttered popcorn, or low-fat desserts. Allow your children to participate in the grocery shopping and cooking so they have an investment in the food you buy and prepare. Finally, be a good role model. If your child sees you opting for an apple instead of an eclair, he or she will be more likely to follow suit.

Excuse #4: "It's too late—I don't feel like cooking. Let's eat out."

Reality: Okay, some of the time. But think how easy it is to eat at home when last night's chicken or pasta is sitting in the refrigerator.

Excuse #5: "There's no food in the house."

Reality: This is an easy one to solve, if you follow my suggestions for food to keep on hand, which requires only a trip to the store from time to time.

GETTING ORGANIZED FOR FAST MEALS

Of course, sitting down with a pencil and pad once a week to plan your week's menu would be an ideal way to approach the issue of bringing cooking back into your life. But, since *not* planning meals ahead is exactly the reason that *fast food* is what's appealing, the planning ahead concept must take on a slightly different meaning: not what you'll cook and when, but what you will keep on hand and what to do with it on the spur of the moment. Keep a piece of paper on or near the refrigerator for jotting down items as you need them. Make at least a mental note of the nights you plan to cook and what you will prepare. A trip to the store once a week will allow you to continue to be spontaneous about cooking, yet it will put you one step closer to making fast food at home a reality.

Once you have developed the following inventory of quick-to-fix food in your kitchen, you can look in your cupboards, refrigerator, and freezer to see what meal you can create. The secret to eating fast and healthy at home for a single person, a couple, or a family, is simplicity. Even if you have but five or ten minutes to fix something to eat, you can make it something good, with or without packaged and take-out meals. Focus on one portion of the meal. There's no need for an array of elaborate dishes. Besides, a one-pot meal saves clean-up time, especially when you use a pot in which a dish can be cooked, served, and stored. You'll find many of my recipes can be made in one pot. If you choose a main dish that is a bit more involved, then serve a simple vegetable on the side. If the main dish is simply chicken or fish that takes little time, prepare a more exciting salad or one of our fried rice dishes. Make use of recommended convenience products— those that sacrifice little, if any, taste or nutrition when time is of the essence.

Start by developing the following inventory of food to keep on hand for quick meals. Then make a list of the many options available with these foods.

FOOD CHECKLIST FOR FAST MEALS AT HOME

Pasta and grains: Any kind of commercially made pasta is quick, but fresh pasta from the deli or freezer case is even quicker—it boils up in a minute or two. Top your favorite pasta with the marinara sauce of your choice. (Our review of sauces follows, page 163.)

Watch for the new precooked no-boil variety of lasagna noodle called Pasta de Fino by de Rosa. They can be simply wetted and layered in a casserole or rolled up with spinach and part-skim ricotta cheese and topped with tomato sauce.

Note: Oil is *not* necessary when cooking pasta, rice, and hot cereals. A little bit of salt will make the dish tastier and the sodium price is not high. Remember ⅛ teaspoon of salt contains 300 milligrams of sodium. That is for the entire *pot* of rice, which fits well into the Fast-Food Diet goal of 3000.

Rice is great for "batch" cooks, who like to do their week's cooking on a Saturday or Sunday afternoon. Brown rice is best, but it takes forty-five minutes to cook, so keep regular rice on hand, which is done in twenty minutes. Uncle Ben's long-grain and wild rice is a staple in my house. Substitute chicken broth for half the water and add garlic instead of salt for variety (1 cup broth has 776 milligrams of sodium, or about 200 milligrams of sodium per half cup cooked rice—a reasonable amount). Minute or "boil-in-a-bag" rice is an option, but texture and flavor are sacrificed.

A pot of rice can be served first time around with chicken, fish, or a stir-fry dish. See ideas on second-time-around rice dishes later in this chapter.

I also keep on hand the Near East products—couscous, tabbouleh, or pilaf mixtures—a nice change from rice and potato. I generally omit the oil, use half the flavor packet, and, during the last five minutes, steam the broccoli by placing it on top of the cooking rice.

Meat, poultry or fish: If these are frozen in your freezer, particularly in individual portions such as breast halves, fillets, or cutlets, you can turn them into a meal in minutes using one of my recipes. Fresh fish cooks very fast, ten minutes per inch. Chicken is easily done in fifteen minutes. Although more expensive, the boneless, skinless chicken breasts save time. Be aware that meat without bones is less flavorful, and a marinade may be perfect for added flavor. Check the teriyaki marinade in Chapter 14 for chicken or a lean flank steak. Some supermarkets offer ready-made kabobs that are easily barbecued without added fat. Look for sliced meats ready for stir-frying.

Fresh vegetables: Buy only the mushrooms, zucchini, broccoli, and salad greens that you plan to use in the first half of the week. Whether they last through the rest of the week depends on how fresh they were when you bought them. Keep less perishable vegetables on hand, including potatoes, carrots, and winter squash.

If time is the reason you skip vegetables, look for prewashed spinach for variety in your salad. Shredded cabbage can be used for salad (see my coleslaw recipe—Green Cabbage Salad) or on sandwiches. Sliced carrots can be eaten plain or tossed in a salad or stir-fry. Some supermarkets offer cut vegetables such as cauliflower, broccoli, and mushrooms, all ready to stir-fry. Pineapples can be purchased peeled and cored, a great time-saver.

Steam vegetables using a collapsible steamer basket placed in a large pot, with one inch of water in the bottom. Cook vegetables just to the crisp-tender stage so they look and taste best and retain more nutrients. Vegetables are naturals for microwaving, which saves time, retains nutrients, and keeps color and flavor at their best.

Minced garlic in a jar is found in the produce section. It's great when you are in a hurry, certainly much better than the powdered types of garlic sprinkle, although I personally feel that the real thing is worth the extra effort.

Frozen vegetables and fruits: Peas and corn and perhaps a piece of fruit or bread can become a meal on those days when you've had a heavy lunch and need only a light snack at dinnertime. Frozen spinach works well in manicotti filling, dips, or soups. Other frozen vegetables, in my opinion, have a hard time competing with flavor and texture of fresh, but they can help you out in a pinch. Nutritionally, they are fine, with only a slight amount of salt—50 milligrams per half cup.

Frozen berries and melon are acceptable with a yogurt topping for breakfast, or added to cereal.

Canned vegetables and fruits: Canned vegetables are generally too great a sacrifice in taste and texture, not to mention their typical sodium content of 242 milligrams per half cup. Canned beans, such as black, kidney, garbanzo, and pinto beans, are great staples to use in salads or in main dishes. Combine beans with leftover rice for a Caribbean-style dish. (See my recipe for Kidney and Garbanzo Bean salad, page 191.) Use the pinto beans for a dip with tortilla chips, or use them as a filling in a tortilla.

Canned water chestnuts, bamboo shoots, and baby corn are rarely sold fresh, and are ideal for additions to last-minute stir-fries. Artichoke hearts and hearts of palm are a nice surprise in a salad. Canned corn and beets can provide a vegetable in a pinch. And what would Thanksgiving be without canned pumpkin?

Although I recommend fresh fruits as much as possible, the few canned varieties that can be tasty include pineapple (especially when used in cooking), cherries, applesauce, pears, and mandarin oranges.

Sauces: Food purists may shun bottled sauces such as spaghetti sauce and barbecue sauce, yet many admit they are mighty handy to have around. These include bottled spaghetti sauces, which are about 130 calories per half cup, including about a teaspoon of oil, salsa, barbecue sauce, horseradish sauce, and various oriental sauces (duck, stir-fry, plum, hoison, etc.). Tastes vary from brand to brand, but the more expensive are generally higher in quality. Pass on the cream-based sauces due to their high saturated-fat content. The Contadina marinara and pesto sauces are wonderful. See the recipe for Pasta with Pesto Sauce, page 220, to make sure you use it in the appropriate amount to keep your meal within the recommended fat guidelines.

Keep whole tomatoes, tomato paste, and tomato sauce on hand for chicken, rice, or other pasta dishes. Tomato paste in a tube is an ingenious new alternative to the can of tomato paste, which is a bit messy when half a can remains.

Jams, jellies, and preserves can be used on breakfast breads. They are a no-fat alternative to butter, margarine, or cream cheese. They can also be used as a base for a sauce.

When choosing sauces, read labels, and choose those with the shortest list of additives. Experiment till you find brands you like, and use them as a condiment or a seasoning, without drenching or heavily coating the pasta, meat, or stir-fry.

Canned soups: You won't find creamed canned soups as ingredients in the Fast-Food Recipes, and for good reason. Most are loaded with sodium, fat, and artificial flavoring. I do, however, recommend the canned chicken or beef broth (Swanson's is an acceptable brand). Although their sodium content is high, they can be used in limited amounts, and their taste is not that significantly different from home-made broth when used with other fresh ingredients in a soup, stew, or sauce.

New, more nutritionally acceptable soups that can be simply re-heated for a last-minute meal are becoming more available. These include the Progresso minestrone, vegetable, chicken noodle, split pea, and lentil.

Bread products: Buy 100 percent whole-grain breads. If, on occasion, you buy sourdough bread or bagels that are sold in a paper bag, be sure to transfer them to a sealed plastic bag for a longer life.

The Pillsbury pizza crust in a can is not a bad stand-in for the real thing. Dust with cornmeal and top with lots of fresh mushrooms, bell peppers, and onion and a bit of Parmesan, Romano, or mozzarella cheese to mask the slightly artificial flavor. See my recipe for Fresh Tomato Pizza for the proportion of ingredients to keep your pizza low in fat. Try the ready-made pizza crust such as Boboli for the instant pizza.* A crusty loaf of sourdough bread can be cut in half lengthwise and turned into a great pizza.

Bridgford frozen ready-to-bake bread dough is also good as pizza crust. Or, it can be shaped into rolls or loaves. Use it to make your own "homemade" cinnamon rolls—with less fat and sugar, and more cinnamon and raisins than store-bought varieties. The aroma of hot baking bread is heartwarming. Try Pillsbury's soft breadsticks.

Corn or flour tortillas can be stuffed with meat, seafood, beans, or vegetables for a quick meal. Buy soft instead of crispy tortillas, which are fried. Heat in a nonstick pan or in a microwave—either way, without added fat. Try my Baked Tortilla Chips for a crunch. Tortillas can be kept frozen and microwaved, steamed, or popped into a toaster oven—no frying necessary.

* I prefer to toast it first, then add hot toppings, to keep the crust crisp—more of a challenge with more vegetables as toppings.

The Pepperidge Farm bread and corn-bread stuffing is good for dressing or casseroles.

Pita bread can be filled with sandwich or salad filling. Cut them in triangles and use them as dippers, as described in Chapter 15 "Party Snacks." If you can find a source at a Greek grocery or restaurant, it will be worth the extra stop. They freeze well, too.

If you have *too much* bread on hand, make a French toast breakfast, according to my recipe in Chapter 10.

Dairy: Keep plain nonfat or low-fat yogurt on hand for smoothies or as a topping on berries or melon. It's a great substitute for sour cream on fish or as a filling in a tortilla. Season with herbs, garlic, or lemon. Use lemon yogurt as a dressing in fruit salad or strawberry yogurt as a pie filling.

Buy shredded mozzarella cheese for quick pizza topping. Freshly grated Parmesan is also available, and is a great improvement over the stuff in cans. Use as quickly as possible, however, since this dries out and spoils faster than cheese in a block.

Keep powdered milk on hand for emergencies, including buttermilk for pancakes. Canned evaporated low-fat or nonfat milk is great for creamed soups, since it is richer than fluid milk, without more fat.

Vinegars: Flavored vinegars are great for last-minute salad dressing when added to a little olive oil. Try balsamic, tarragon, champagne, or raspberry vinegars.

Oils and salad dressings: Keep two basic oils on hand: olive oil and nonflavored low saturated-fat vegetable oil. I suggest Puritan since it is made from canola oil, the least saturated oil available. Both oils are high in monounsaturated fat, and this combination is cardio-protective. Try making your own salad dressing with various combinations of vinegars and oils; I provide recipes to help with this in Chapter 12. As for the prepared salad dressings, clear or oil-based dressings are generally better choices than cream-based varieties. There are many oil-free dressings available, containing less than 10 calories per ounce; reduced-calorie varieties may have a third less calories than their higher-calorie counterparts. Check labels and experiment until you find one you like.

The nonstick vegetable sprays, such as Pam, are great for less fat and calories in the skillet, sauté pan, and casserole dish. Olive oil Pam can be used on vegetables or when a stronger flavor is desired. Use butter-flavored Pam on corn-on-the-cob or popcorn.

Seasonings and herbs: The most common seasonings used in the Fast-Food Recipes are garlic, onion, lemon, vinegar, wine, reduced-sodium soy sauce, and Dijon mustard. I have suggested salt and pepper "to taste" in many recipes. Of course, there is no need to add the salt if your taste buds have been trained not to require it. Keep spices simple. Too many spices confuse the palate. When you put too many spices in too many dishes, they all begin to taste the same. The recipes will guide you, along with your own palate. The following list summarizes the food to have on hand.

Food Checklist for Fast Meals at Home

Pasta: fresh, deli, or dried

Rice: white, brown, regular, or quick-cooking

Boxed rice products: couscous, tabbouleh, pilaf

Meat, poultry, fish

Fresh vegetables:

    limit perishables to amount to be used in near future: mushrooms, zucchini, broccoli, and salad greens. Keep on hand less perishable produce: potatoes, carrots, winter squash.

Minced garlic in a jar

Frozen vegetables and fruits: peas, corn, spinach; berries, melon

Canned vegetables and fruits:

    black, kidney, garbanzo, and pinto beans

    water chestnuts, bamboo shoots, baby corn, artichoke hearts, hearts of palm;

    pineapple, cherries, applesauce, pears, mandarin oranges

Sauces:

    spaghetti sauces (marinara or pesto), salsa, barbecue sauce, horseradish sauce, oriental sauces

    whole tomatoes, tomato paste, tomato sauce

    jams, jellies, preserves

Canned soups:

    chicken or beef broth

    Progresso minestrone, vegetable, chicken noodle, split pea, lentil

Bread products:

    bread, bagels, rolls, pita

    pizza dough

    frozen bread dough

    corn or flour tortillas

Dairy:
   yogurt: plain, nonfat, or low-fat
   yogurt, fruited: nonfat, or low-fat
   cheese: mozzarella, parmesan, or other low-fat cheeses
   milk: fluid, powdered or canned evaporated
Vinegar, seasoned
Oils:
   olive oil
   Puritan
   salad dressing: fat free, reduced calorie, or oil-based dressing
   vegetable spray
Seasonings and herbs:
   garlic, onion, lemon, vinegar, wine, reduced-sodium soy sauce,
   Dijon mustard, salt, pepper

COOKING METHODS THAT SAVE TIME

Timesaving cooking methods include a microwave oven, toaster oven, as well as simple, stove-top cooking in place of oven methods. Fish is the fastest-cooking animal protein, with chicken and beef right behind. The stir-fry method is quick with or without meat, and you need not use a wok; a nonstick pan will do. The rule is high temperature, short time when stir-frying. Stick to vegetables that cook fast if you are really in a hurry. Refer to suggestions in the recipes ahead.

Microwaving is great for vegetables and fish, not so good for pasta or rice, and great for reheating all foods. The advantage of microwaving, in addition to faster cooking time, is that you don't need to add fat to meat, chicken or fish.

Although roasts, stews, and casseroles take longer to cook, they require very little of *your* time for preparation. My Chicken Pot Roast with Rosemary and Garlic (page 210), for example, need only be put in a pot along with potatoes, carrots, and a few seasonings. But it takes longer to roast in the oven than the Cajun Chicken (page 210), which is prepared on the stove top or barbecue. Consider your own time situation. Slow cookers, or crockpots can be filled with a stew in the morning, and will be done when you get home.

Barbecuing on a rack over coals is fun, and low in fat, since you need not add any fat to cook. Trim fat from meat to prevent flare-up of flames and to reduce calories. Check my recipes for marinades and sauces.

MAKING TWO MEALS OUT OF ONE

When you do take the time to cook, make your efforts really worthwhile. A basic rule of cooking, whether it's for one or two or more, is to cook for more than one meal each time you cook. These "planned leftovers" can be quickly served in new ways. Here is a list of "extras" that provide the basis for another meal, allowing you to turn one meal into two with little extra work.

- Extra pancakes, French toast, muffins, or even oatmeal, left over from the weekend can be reheated during the week.
- Sandwich fillings, such as tuna or chicken salad, can be made in enough quantity to provide two or three days of brown bags.
- Whenever you make a salad, clean all your greens, the entire head of broccoli, the whole bag of carrots, et cetera, even if you don't intend to use them all. Just store in seal-tight plastic bags or containers, and the next salad will come much easier.
- When you need just a half onion, cut up the whole onion, store in a plastic bag, and use the rest later.
- Steam more vegetables than you plan to eat. Use extras as cold snacks or in salads. Puree leftover vegetables in a blender or food processor and add milk for a "soup." This works great with broccoli (see my Pureed Broccoli Soup recipe, page 195), as well as cauliflower and corn. Enjoy with a roll or a slice of whole-grain bread, toasted if you like. If you feel ambitious, mix up a batch of corn bread (boxed mixes make it easy), and your leftover vegetable puree is turned into a delightful meal.
- Soups are easy to make in extra quantities, and a great way to use up leftover pasta and vegetables. Freeze the amount you don't intend to eat over the next several days.
- Prepare extra chicken breasts for sandwiches, lunches, or tortilla stuffers. Toss chicken into pasta or rice dishes, or use in a salad.
- Cook extra burgers. Reheat in the microwave for another meal. Eating burgers at home instead of out is a great way to satisfy an old craving without all the fat that might be in a burger prepared at a restaurant; and it's such an easy meal!
- Extra fish is great in sandwiches or tortillas.
- Pasta dishes are great reheated. To store any pasta that is left over, cover with cold water and refrigerate, or add any sauce to prevent it from becoming a congealed mass. It'll be ready for tomorrow's lunch or dinner.
- Cook extra rice to turn into "fried rice," according to my recipes in Chapter 14.

• Potatoes that have been steamed or baked can be turned into fries, or mashed and mixed with cabbage, or added to corn chowder soup—or any other soup. Cook double the amount you plan to eat, and refer to my recipe calling for leftover baked potatoes (page 228), called Potato Fries. You won't even miss McDonald's french fries after these!

FREEZING FOOD

If you do get into the habit of cooking extra food, you may find you want to freeze food occasionally. There is nothing better than the opportunity to "heat and eat" a home-cooked meal on the night when you truly don't feel like cooking. Here is a list of fast foods that freeze well, without wrecking their texture or consistency.

Foods that Freeze Well

Red meat and chicken

Raw shrimp and scallops (other fish can be frozen, but their quality suffers)

Soups

Pureed cooked vegetables

Blanched vegetables and fruit (the heat in blanching destroys enzyme action that causes deterioration)

Hard cheeses

Flour, all kinds (keeps bugs out if you don't use it too often)

Breads, muffins, cookies, pies, cakes

Nuts and dried fruits

Pancakes, French toast

Leftover rice

Butter, margarine

Coffee

Chopped onions and green pepper

Partially used containers of olives, pimentos, water chestnuts, and bamboo shoots

Fresh ginger

Fresh mushrooms, sliced or whole

Bananas, whole with peel or peeled and sliced for use in smoothies or Puree of Frozen Banana

Tomato-based sauces

Foods that Do 🖙 Not Freeze Well

Cooked pasta

Yogurt, sour cream, and cottage cheese

Melons

Eggs

Potatoes

Custards and creams

Mayonnaise

Raw tomatoes and most other raw vegetables (blanch first)

FAST-FOOD-AT-HOME RECIPE COLLECTION

The Fast-Food-at-Home Recipe Collection was developed in my kitchen. These recipes actually preceded the diet. I was motivated to develop them by the scores of busy and active people I counsel as a registered dietitian in San Diego. My clients were looking for ways to combine healthy eating habits with their time-demanding careers. I soon saw the need for quickly prepared meals and snacks—healthy ones.

You will find many of your favorite fast foods reborn here, healthier versions of the old, such as chicken tacos, pizza, and burgers with less fat, calories, and preparation time.

If just the *idea* of cooking turns you off, choose the recipes or "food ideas" that require "assembling" rather than "cooking." Many of these take only a few minutes to prepare.

The recipes reflect my philosophy that healthy food can taste great and be easy to prepare. Because my background is nutrition and not professional cooking, the recipes and methods are without roots in traditions of cookery that add too much fat and calories. Each recipe is followed by vital information on calories and what percentage of those calories are in carbohydrate, protein, fat, and the amount of fat, cholesterol, saturated fat, sodium, and fiber per serving.

Modifications Used in Fast-Food Recipes

The Fast-Food Recipes have been modified to score in the upper end of the Fast-Food Rating Scale. They emphasize light, fresh, and simple. Here are a few of the recipe substitutions I've used. You may want to use these, as well, to adapt your old favorites.

Food	Instead of	Use	Calories Saved
French Toast	2 eggs	1 egg + 1 egg white	40
Cheese and Crackers	3 oz. Cheddar or jack cheese	3 oz. part-skim mozzarella	120
Barbecued Teriyaki Flank Steak	3 oz. sirloin chunk or ribs	3 oz. flank or round	300
Puree of Frozen Banana (ice cream)	½ c. regular ice cream	½ c. frozen bananas	75
Pasta Primavera	2 c. w/alfredo sauce	2 c. w/chicken broth thickened w/ cornstarch	400
Cuban-style Beef in Tortilla	3 oz. ground beef	3 oz. ground turkey	100
	2 T. sour cream	2 T. plain yogurt	55
Potato Fries	3 oz. french fries	3 oz. baked potato	180
Barbecued Chicken Breasts with Tabasco and Lime	3 oz. dark meat chicken w/skin	3 oz. light, skinless in our sauce	100

You will notice that the recipes have been adapted and, in some cases, presented in combination with other foods in order to show how they can meet the 30 percent–fat criteria. For example, the Orange-Vinaigrette Dressing with less than 20 calories per tablespoon can, when calculated alone, yield 90 percent of calories from fat. It would be misleading, however, to suggest that this is not a wise food choice, because it can still be included with an entire day's food plan that has no more than 30 percent of the total day's calories from fat.

These recipes are tried and true and have been well received by all, making it unnecessary to cook separate meals for other family members. Many of the recipes also transport well in brown bags, offering food solutions for the next day's lunch.

Remember, food is your body's only fuel. Make it fast, but make it efficient.

CHAPTER · 10

BREAKFASTS

Yes, you are doing great to gobble down your cereal or a piece of toast on a weekday morning, and I commend you. But if, on the weekend, you are in the mood for a change of pace, make it brunch, at home. Take advantage of the opportunity to *stay home* and enjoy a leisurely meal, without the traditional breakfast of bacon and eggs.

 French Toast with Fresh Fruit Sauce

Oatcakes with Applesauce

Scrambled Eggs with Spinach in a Pita

Orange-Banana Smoothie

Oatmeal with Cinnamon, Raisins, and Brown Sugar

Oatmeal-Blueberry Muffins

Wheat Bran Muffins with Raisins

FRENCH TOAST WITH FRESH FRUIT SAUCE

1 slice Fast-Food French Toast provides:
80 calories
58% carbohydrate
20% protein
22% fat
2 g fat
46 mg cholesterol
0.4 g saturated fat
181 mg sodium
1.8 g fiber

1 slice traditional French toast recipe made with white bread provides:
153 calories
45% carbohydrate
15% protein
40% fat
7 g fat
60 mg cholesterol
2.8 g saturated fat
257 mg sodium
<1 g fiber

1 whole egg
1 egg white
2 tablespoons nonfat or low-fat milk
6 slices whole wheat bread
½ teaspoon ground cinnamon

1 Heat a large nonstick skillet on the stove.
2 In a pie pan or bowl, combine the egg, egg white, and milk.
3 Soak the bread in the mixture, turning to coat on both sides.
4 Sprinkle with cinnamon.
5 Cook in the skillet over medium heat for about 3 minutes on each side, or until golden brown.

NOTE: Calorie and fiber values vary with different breads. Although calories may go up with heartier breads, it's worth the price, because vitamins, minerals, and fiber also increase.

Makes 6 slices

 # FRESH FRUIT SAUCE

⅓ cup Fresh Fruit Sauce provides:
70 calories
93% carbohydrate
5% protein
3% fat
0 g fat
0 mg cholesterol
0 g saturated fat
1.4 mg sodium
0.4 g fiber

⅓ cup maple syrup provides:
252 calories
100% carbohydrate
0% protein
0% fat
0 g fat
0 mg cholesterol
0 g saturated fat
10 mg sodium
0 g fiber

¼ cup water
¼ cup raisins
1 ripe banana, cut up
1 orange, peeled and quartered
Juice of 1 lemon

1 Put the water in a saucepan and add the raisins. Bring to a boil.
2 Puree the banana and orange in a food processor or blender.
3 Add the raisin-water and lemon mixture to the puree.
4 Serve on French toast or pancakes.

NOTE: The Fresh Fruit Sauce provides a good source of vitamins A and C, as well as potassium and other micronutrients—a considerable advantage over the maple syrup.

Makes 4 servings

OATCAKES WITH APPLESAUCE

1 Oatcake provides:
110 calories
64% carbohydrate
21% protein
15% fat
2 g fat
40 mg cholesterol
0.3 g saturated fat
155 mg sodium
2.4 g fiber

1 pancake from a mix, prepared according to instructions:
120 calories
58% carbohydrate
13% protein
29% fat
4 g fat
40 mg cholesterol
1 g saturated fat
320 mg sodium
0 g fiber

1½ cups nonfat milk or buttermilk, divided

1 cup quick or regular rolled oats

1 whole egg, or 2 egg whites

½ cup whole wheat flour

1 tablespoon brown sugar

1 teaspoon baking powder

¼ teaspoon salt

1 Combine ½ cup milk and oats in a bowl. (Old-fashioned oats require a little more soaking, about 5 minutes.)

2 Add 1 cup milk and the egg or whites and mix well.

3 Stir in the dry ingredients only till moistened.

4 Cook on a hot nonstick griddle, using ¼ cup of batter for each pancake, turning when the top is bubbly and edges slightly dry.

5 Serve with applesauce.

NOTE: These delicious and hearty pancakes require slightly longer baking than regular pancakes.

Makes seven 5-inch pancakes

 # SCRAMBLED EGGS WITH SPINACH IN A PITA

1 6-inch pita and ½ cup Scrambled Eggs provides:
210 calories
44% carbohydrate
27% protein
28% fat
6 g fat
275 mg cholesterol
1.9 g saturated fat
348 mg sodium
0.5 g fiber

2 whole eggs

2 egg whites

2 tablespoons nonfat or low-fat milk

6 leaves raw spinach, chopped (frozen spinach can be substituted)

2 scallions, chopped

Pepper to taste

Grated Parmesan cheese to taste

2 whole wheat pita breads

1 Combine all the ingredients except the pita in a bowl.
2 Scramble in a nonstick skillet.
3 Cut each pita in half. Heat in toaster and fill each pita with the eggs.
Enjoy.

Makes 2 servings

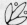 # ORANGE-BANANA SMOOTHIE

1 cup plain nonfat yogurt
1 ripe banana, cut into pieces
1 orange, peeled and quartered
Honey (optional), to taste

1 In a blender container, combine all the ingredients.
2 Cover, blend until smooth.

NOTE: Makes a terrific accompaniment to pancakes, French toast, or just plain peanut butter on toast.

Makes 2 servings

OATMEAL WITH CINNAMON, RAISINS, AND BROWN SUGAR

A ⅔ cup serving of cooked oats plus 2 teaspoons raisins provides:
114 calories
73% carbohydrate
14% protein
12% fat
1.5 g fat
0 mg cholesterol
0.3 g saturated fat
1.3 mg sodium
1.9 g fiber

1½ cups water
¼ teaspoon salt (optional)
⅔ cup rolled oats
2 teaspoons raisins
Dash ground cinnamon
Dash brown sugar

1 Bring the water and salt, if desired, to a boil in a pot.
2 Stir the oats and raisins into the briskly boiling water.
3 Cook for 5 minutes or longer, stirring occasionally.
4 Place in a serving bowl and sprinkle with cinnamon and brown sugar.

NOTE: Although oatmeal is a good source of fiber, we cannot rely on it (or any other *single* food) to meet our daily need of 15 to 20 grams. Choose high-fiber foods all day long, and don't forget fruits and vegetables.

Makes 2 servings

OATMEAL-BLUEBERRY MUFFINS

1 muffin provides:
168 calories
58% carbohydrate
9% protein
32% fat
6 g fat
24 mg cholesterol
1.0 g saturated fat
182 mg sodium
1.6 g fiber

1¼ cups rolled oats
1¼ cups flour
⅓ cup plus 2 tablespoons sugar
1 tablespoon baking powder
½ teaspoon salt
1 cup nonfat or low-fat milk
¼ cup vegetable oil
1 egg, beaten
¾ cup frozen blueberries
2 teaspoons ground cinnamon

1 Preheat the oven to 425°.

2 Combine the oats, flour, ⅓ cup sugar, baking powder, and salt in a large bowl; mix well.

3 Mix the milk, oil, and egg in another bowl. Add to the oatmeal mixture and stir until just moistened.

4 Fold in the blueberries.

5 Spoon the batter into muffin cups, about three-quarters full, and bake for about 15 minutes, until muffins are golden brown and a toothpick inserted in center comes out clean.

6 Dust with the 2 tablespoons sugar and the cinnamon.

NOTE: This muffin is not only lower in fat than the muffin you buy at the bakery, it's also likely to be smaller in size.

Makes 12 muffins

WHEAT BRAN MUFFINS WITH RAISINS

1 muffin provides:
172 calories
69% carbohydrate
7% protein
24% fat
5 g fat
0.1 mg cholesterol
0.6 g saturated fat
156 mg sodium
1.6 g fiber

1¼ cups flour

1 cup bran or wheat flakes cereal

⅔ cup sugar

2½ teaspoons baking powder

¼ teaspoon salt

½ teaspoon ground cinnamon

½ cup nonfat milk

¼ cup Puritan oil (or other unflavored salad oil)

2 egg whites, lightly beaten

¾ cup raisins

1 Preheat the oven to 425°.

2 Combine the dry ingredients in a large bowl and mix well.

3 Mix the wet ingredients in another bowl. Add to the dry ingredients and stir until just moistened.

4 Fold in the raisins.

5 Spoon the batter into muffin cups, about three-quarters full, and bake for about 15 minutes, until toothpick inserted in center comes out clean.

(*continued on next page*)

NOTE: With all the talk about the benefits of oat bran and the soluble fibers lowering cholesterol, it's easy to forget the benefit of the first-popular wheat bran, which has a higher water-absorbing quality than oat bran, and thus, may provide added bulk to stools when needed.

Makes 12 muffins

CHAPTER 11

BROWN-BAG LUNCHES

Before you decide that you don't need a recipe for such brown-bag fillers as tuna salad or, much less, cheese and crackers, look again. I have modified those favorite foods to save you fat and calories, to make them the very best they can be, without compromising flavor or the nutritional quality of your diet.

 Tuna Salad on Whole Wheat

Avocado and Swiss Cheese Sandwich

Revised Peanut Butter and Jelly Sandwich

Lox, Cream Cheese, and Bagel

Cheese and Crackers

Bean Nut Butter Sandwich

Pinto Bean Burrito

Chicken Taco

French Bread Stuffed with Tomato Sauce, Zucchini, and Cheese

Light Cream Cheese on Toast with Cucumbers

TUNA SALAD ON WHOLE WHEAT

1 Fast-Food Tuna sandwich provides:
260 calories
40% carbohydrate
44% protein
16% fat
4.5 g fat
30 mg cholesterol
0.3 g saturated fat
679 mg sodium
7.6 g fiber

1 deli tuna sandwich (typically prepared) provides:
480 calories
26% carbohydrate
29% protein
45% fat
24 g fat
68 mg cholesterol
4.5 g saturated fat
756 mg sodium
7.6 g fiber

1-ounce can water-packed tuna, drained
2 tablespoons plain lowfat yogurt or low-calorie mayonnaise
¼ cup chopped celery
1 scallion, sliced
¼ cup chopped vegetables (carrots, zucchini, broccoli, mushrooms)
4 slices whole wheat bread
2 tomatoes, sliced
Lettuce leaves

1 Combine the tuna and yogurt or mayonnaise in a bowl.
2 Blend in the vegetables.
3 Spread the salad on the bread; top with tomato and lettuce.

Makes 2 sandwiches

 # AVOCADO AND SWISS CHEESE SANDWICH

1 Avocado and Swiss Sandwich provides:
246 calories
42% carbohydrate
20% protein
38% fat
11 g fat
16 mg cholesterol
3.7 g saturated fat
521 mg sodium
7.1 g fiber

⅛ avocado, peeled and sliced
1 ounce lite Swiss cheese
1 teaspoon mustard
Tomato slices
Onion slices
Bell pepper rings
Cucumber slices
2 slices whole wheat bread

Assemble sandwich and enjoy.

NOTE: Good source of fiber.

Makes 1 sandwich

REVISED PEANUT BUTTER AND JELLY SANDWICH

1 Revised Peanut Butter and Jelly Sandwich provides:
245 calories
50% carbohydrate
14% protein
36% fat
10 g fat
0 mg cholesterol
1.8 g saturated fat
334 mg sodium
2.7 g fiber

1 peanut butter and jelly sandwich (2 tablespoons peanut butter, 2 teaspoons jelly) provides:
356 calories
41% carbohydrate
14% protein
45% fat
18 g fat
0 mg cholesterol
3.1 g saturated fat
410 mg sodium
4.1 g fiber

1 tablespoon peanut butter
1 teaspoon jelly
2 slices wheat bread

Assemble your sandwich and enjoy.

NOTE: The usual peanut butter sandwich uses double the amount of peanut butter and jelly.

Makes 1 sandwich

LOX, CREAM CHEESE, AND BAGEL

1 Bagel Sandwich provides:
296 calories
31% carbohydrate
26% protein
31% fat
10 g fat
22 mg cholesterol
0.7 g saturated fat
205 mg sodium
0.5 g fiber

1 whole wheat bagel
2 ounces lox
2 teaspoons cream cheese
Onion slice

Assemble sandwich and enjoy.

Makes 1 serving

1 bagel with 2 tablespoons cream cheese, 2 ounces lox provides:
393 calories
33% carbohydrate
22% protein
45% fat
19.5 g fat
53 mg cholesterol
6.9 g saturated fat
288 mg sodium
0.5 g fiber

CHEESE AND CRACKERS

2 triple RyKrisp crackers and 1 ounce mozzarella cheese provide:

118 calories
36% carbohydrate
28% protein
36% fat
5 g fat
16 mg cholesterol
2.9 g saturated fat
245 mg sodium
1.6 g fiber

16 Wheat Thins and 1 ounce cheddar cheese provide:

258 calories
32% carbohydrate
15% protein
53% fat
15 g fat
29 mg cholesterol
6.0 g saturated fat
176 mg sodium
0 g fiber

NO-FAT CRACKERS:

Finn Crisp

Flat bread

Hardtack

Wasa Crackers

LOW-FAT CRACKERS:

Ak-Mak

Breadsticks

Melba toast

RyKrisp

Oyster crackers

Saltines

Canadian stone ground

1 Choose crackers from the categories above.

2 Accompany with low-fat spreads, low-fat cheese slices, or fresh fruit.

 # BEAN NUT BUTTER SANDWICH

1-inch pita bread and ¼ cup bean mixture provide:

234 calories
71% carbohydrate
18% protein
11% fat
3 g fat
0.3 mg cholesterol
0 g saturated fat
729 mg sodium
6.6 g fiber

1 16-ounce can garbanzo beans, drained

¼ cup nonfat plain yogurt or light mayonnaise

1 tablespoon Dijon mustard

Crackers or whole wheat pita bread

Tomato slices

Lettuce leaves

1 Put the beans, yogurt or mayonnaise, and mustard in a food processor or blender and puree until smooth.

2 Serve on crackers or pita bread with tomato and lettuce.

NOTE: This sandwich is high in fiber and a good source of iron.

Makes 6 servings or 1½ cups

PINTO BEAN BURRITO

1 Fast-Food Diet Burrito provides:
205 calories
73% carbohydrate
16% protein
11% fat
3 g fat
0 mg cholesterol
0.1 g saturated fat
67 mg sodium
4.5 g fiber

1 Bean Burrito at Taco Bell provides:
350 calories
62% carbohydrate
15% protein
26% fat
10 g fat
9 mg cholesterol
3.0 g saturated fat
763 mg sodium
4.5 g fiber

⅓ cup canned or fresh cooked pinto beans
1 flour tortilla
1 tomato, sliced
1 tablespoon chopped onion
1 tablespoon salsa

1 Place the beans in the tortilla.
2 Add the tomato, onion, and salsa.
3 Wrap in plastic wrap and microwave until warm, about 1 to 2 minutes.
4 If not using a microwave, heat the beans in a saucepan, and warm the tortilla in a nonstick pan, then assemble.

NOTE: This meal is a good source of fiber.

Makes 1 burrito

CHICKEN TACO

1 Fast-Food Diet Taco provides:
318 calories
31% carbohydrate
50% protein
19% fat
7 g fat
96 mg cholesterol
1.2 g saturated fat
391 mg sodium
1.0 g fiber

1 Taco Light from Taco Bell provides:
410 calories
18% carbohydrate
19% protein
63% fat
29 g fat
56 mg cholesterol
12.0 g saturated fat
594 mg sodium
1.0 g fiber.

1 cooked chicken breast (from last night's dinner)
1 corn tortilla
1 tomato, chopped
1 scallion, chopped
Chopped cilantro
2 ounces salsa
2 tablespoons nonfat plain yogurt

1 Skin the chicken if not already done and remove from the bone. Shred meat, if needed.
2 Warm the tortilla in a microwave or nonstick pan (no fat necessary).
3 Place in the tortilla: chicken, tomatoes, scallion, and cilantro. Season with salsa and nonfat yogurt.
4 When packing the taco into a brown-bag lunch, heat the tortilla and chicken in the office microwave before adding the garnishes.

(continued on next page)

NOTE: For a great variation, substitute leftover fish for the chicken, and top with a squeeze of lemon and shredded cabbage instead of tomato and scallion.

Makes 1 taco

FRENCH BREAD STUFFED WITH TOMATO SAUCE, ZUCCHINI, AND CHEESE

⅓ loaf provides:
292 calories
59% carbohydrate
21% protein
20% fat
6.5 g fat
165 mg cholesterol
3.1 g saturated fat
441 mg sodium
3.2 g fiber

FILLING:
1 teaspoon olive oil
2 cups chopped zucchini
1 onion, chopped
1 green bell pepper, chopped
1 red bell pepper, chopped
Chopped fresh basil
3 ounces mozzarella cheese

1 loaf sourdough bread

1 In a nonstick skillet heat the oil and sauté the filling ingredients.
2 Cut the bread in half lengthwise and stuff with the vegetable sauté.
3 Wrap the bread in aluminum foil and bake for 15 minutes at 425°, or take to a picnic or barbecue for an easy dinner with a bottle of California Chardonnay.

Makes 3 servings

LIGHT CREAM CHEESE ON TOAST WITH CUCUMBERS

1 open-faced sandwich provides:
100 calories
56% carbohydrate
13% protein
30% fat
3 g fat
5.5 mg cholesterol
1.2 g saturated fat
169 mg sodium
2.7 g fiber

1 slice whole wheat bread
2 teaspoons light cream cheese
Cucumber slices
Black pepper to taste

1 Toast the bread.
2 Top with the cream cheese and cucumbers, season with pepper, and enjoy.

Makes 1 serving

CHAPTER · 12

SALADS AND SALAD DRESSINGS

If the idea of making a salad is enough to make you call out for a pizza, then simplify. Begin at the store with buying only the amount of fresh produce you will actually use in a week. Then make simple salads with three, two, or even one ingredient. Remember, you are trying to increase your vegetable intake without significantly increasing your fat intake. Salads also give you crunch, and the dressing gives your taste buds the tangy experience, essential to ultimate satisfaction after a meal.

Nutritional analysis of salads shows that they have a high percentage of fat. In some cases, it is because only 25 calories of vegetable or salad greens is topped with 45 calories of dressing, which is okay, but it makes a total of 70 calories with 45 fat calories or 5 grams of fat. That equals 64 percent of calories from fat, too high for a meal or a day, but okay if it is mixed in with the right meal or day. Check your intake of fat grams for the day and compare it to the suggested daily fat intake listed on the chart on page 17.

Step back and take a look at the total picture: you can afford 5 grams of fat in the context of a full meal. But making the salad huge and eating it as your entrée may be a mistake, since three cups of vegetables may still only be 75 calories of vegetables, while a comparable increase of the same salad dressing is 135 calories. And chances are, a large salad has other fat ingredients, such as meat, cheese, seeds, nuts, olives—without the roll that provides the complex carbohydrate. The heartier salads with bean and pasta work out better as entrées, particularly when added oil is limited, because the starch is part of the salads without adding more fat calories. These salads are also perfect for next day's brown bag.

BASIC TOSSED GREEN SALAD WITH VINAIGRETTE

1 serving provides:
97 calories
17% carbohydrate
4% protein
79% fat
9 g fat
0 mg cholesterol
1.3 g saturated fat
4.6 mg sodium
0.7 g fiber

VINAIGRETTE:

2 teaspoons olive oil

1 clove garlic, crushed

1 tablespoon red wine vinegar, preferably balsamic

¼ teaspoon sugar, honey, or artificial sweetener

Juice of ½ lemon

2 cups salad greens

1 Mix the vinaigrette ingredients together.

2 Toss the dressing with the salad greens.

SERVING SUGGESTIONS: Use romaine green leaves, toss in grated Parmesan cheese, and top with homemade garlic croutons (1 slice whole wheat bread, toasted with 1 teaspoon margarine and a sprinkle of garlic powder).

Makes 2 servings

GREENS WITH RED ONION AND CITRUS

1 cup greens with 1 tablespoon Vinaigrette Dressing provides:
59 calories
66% carbohydrate
9% protein
25% fat
2 g fat
0 mg cholesterol
0.2 g saturated fat
3.3 mg sodium
2.3 g fiber

1 cup greens with 1 tablespoon blue cheese dressing provides:
119 calories
35% carbohydrate
7% protein
58% fat
8 g fat
9 mg cholesterol
1.5 g saturated fat
170 mg sodium
2.3 g fiber

ORANGE-VINAIGRETTE DRESSING

1 cup rice vinegar or other mild vinegar

1–2 cloves garlic, minced or mashed

2 tablespoons frozen orange juice

2 tablespoons olive oil

½ teaspoon freshly ground or coarsely ground black
  pepper

2 heads butter lettuce, torn into bite-size pieces

3 oranges, peeled and sectioned

1 small red onion, thinly sliced into rings

1 Combine the dressing ingredients and mix well.

2 Combine the lettuce, oranges, and red onion.

3 Toss all the ingredients with ⅓ cup of the dressing. (Save any remaining dressing for use again.)

Makes 6 1-cup servings

SALAD GREENS WITH AVOCADO AND RAISINS

One cup provides:
57 calories
39% carbohydrate
8% protein
53% fat
4 g fat
0 mg cholesterol
0.5 g saturated fat
9 mg sodium
1.7 g fiber

¼ avocado, peeled and cubed

1 head green leaf lettuce, washed and separated

2 tablespoons raisins

½ cup sliced mushrooms

1 tomato, sliced

DRESSING:

1 tablespoon tarragon vinegar

1 tablespoon olive oil

1 Combine the salad ingredients; toss.

2 Combine the dressing ingredients and season the salad with them.

Makes 4 cups

MARINATED CUCUMBER SLICES

½ cucumber with marinade provides:

15 calories
91% carbohydrate
6% protein
3% fat
0 g fat
0 mg cholesterol
0 g saturated fat
1.4 mg sodium
0.8 g fiber

1 cucumber, sliced
1 scallion, chopped (optional)

MARINADE:
½ cup vinegar, preferably a mild vinegar such as rice or tarragon
½ cup water
1 teaspoon sugar
Freshly ground black pepper to taste

Combine all ingredients for marinade in a bowl; add cucumber and salad to marinade.

Makes approximately 2 cups sliced cucumber, depending on size of cucumber

CUCUMBER, TOMATO, AND FETA CHEESE WITH PINEAPPLE VINEGAR

1 serving provides:
119 calories
38% carbohydrate
18% protein
44% fat
6.5 g fat
25 mg cholesterol
4.4 g saturated fat
333 mg sodium
4.2 g fiber

1 cucumber, chopped
2 tomatoes, chopped
2 ounces feta cheese, crumbled
¼ cup pineapple or other flavored vinegar

1 Combine all ingredients in a bowl.

Makes 2 servings

TOMATO SLICES WITH ASPARAGUS AND DIJON VINAIGRETTE

1 serving provides:
117 calories
34% carbohydrate
13% protein
53% fat
7.5 g fat
0 mg cholesterol
1.0 g saturated fat
80 mg sodium
3.5 g fiber

2 tomatoes, sliced
½ pound asparagus, trimmed, steamed, and cooled

VINAIGRETTE:
1 tablespoon Puritan oil
1 tablespoon vinegar, preferably a wine or champagne
    vinegar
2 teaspoons Dijon mustard

1 Arrange tomatoes and asparagus on a plate.
2 Combine vinaigrette ingredients and drizzle over vegetables.

Makes 2 servings of 1 tomato and ⅔ cup asparagus pieces

CUCUMBER, TOMATO, AND ONION SALAD WITH CREAMY DRESSING

¾ cup provides:
38 calories
68% carbohydrate
13% protein
19% fat
1 g fat
0.9 mg cholesterol
0.1 g saturated fat
12 mg sodium
2.1 g fiber

1 cucumber, cut into ½"-squares
2 tomatoes, cut into ½"-square chunks
3 scallions, sliced

DRESSING:
2 teaspoons light mayonnaise
2 tablespoons nonfat or low-fat plain yogurt
1 tablespoon seasoned vinegar
1 teaspoon honey or sugar, or artificial sweetener to
    taste

1 Combine the vegetables in a bowl.
2 Combine the dressing ingredients and toss with the vegetables.

Makes 4 1-cup servings

GREEN CABBAGE SALAD

1 cup provides:
86 calories
42% carbohydrate
10% protein
48% fat
5 g fat
6 mg cholesterol
0 g saturated fat
47 mg sodium
2.2 g fiber

DRESSING:

1 teaspoon sugar

Salt

1 tablespoon white wine vinegar

2 teaspoons Dijon-style mustard

½ cup nonfat or low-fat plain yogurt

½ cup light mayonnaise

1 medium head green cabbage, cored and shredded

1 carrot, grated

1 small white onion, minced

1 To make the dressing, dissolve the sugar in the vinegar. Whisk in the mustard, yogurt and mayonnaise.

2 Combine all the salad vegetables, and toss them with enough of the dressing to thoroughly coat them. Refrigerate. Keeps covered for up to 1 week.

Makes 7 cups

KIDNEY AND GARBANZO BEANS WITH CAULIFLOWER

½ cup provides:
140 calories
56% carbohydrate
21% protein
24% fat
4 g fat
2.5 mg cholesterol
0.1 g saturated fat
457 mg sodium
6.0 g fiber

1 16-ounce can red kidney beans

1 15-ounce can garbanzo beans

1 small head cauliflower, separated into florets (about 1 cup)

1 small onion, chopped

Fresh parsley or cilantro, chopped

1 tablespoon olive oil

¼ cup grated Parmesan cheese

¼ cup wine vinegar

1 teaspoon coarsely ground black pepper

(*continued on next page*)

1 Drain and rinse the beans.
2 Combine all the ingredients in a bowl.
3 Chill; stir to blend flavors.

Makes 4 cups

 # PASTA SALAD WITH ARTICHOKES AND BASIL

½ cup Pasta Salad provides:
71 calories
54% carbohydrate
14% protein
32% fat
3 g fat
9.4 mg cholesterol
0.8 g saturated fat
70 mg sodium
1.4 g fiber

2 tomatoes, cut into wedges

1 zucchini, sliced

¼ cup (about 10) medium-size pitted black olives

1 medium red onion, chopped

1 ounce feta cheese, crumbled

1 cup cooked rotelle or spiral

6 ounces marinated artichokes, plus 2 teaspoons
   marinade (discard remaining marinade)

¼ cup wine vinegar

2 tablespoons chopped fresh basil, or 1 tablespoon
   dried

Freshly ground black pepper

1 Combine the tomatoes and zucchini with the olives, onion, feta cheese, and pasta.
2 Toss with the artichoke hearts and marinade, vinegar, basil, and pepper to taste.
3 Chill to blend the flavors.

Makes 8 ½-cup servings

SNOW PEA, YELLOW BELL PEPPER, AND MUSHROOM SALAD

1 cup provides:
65 calories
65% carbohydrate
16% protein
19% fat
2 g fat
0 mg cholesterol
0.2 g saturated fat
65 mg sodium
4.5 g fiber

DRESSING:

1 teaspoon sesame oil

1 teaspoon vegetable oil

3 tablespoons white wine vinegar

1 tablespoon sugar, honey, or artificial sweetener

⅛ teaspoon salt

1 teaspoon freshly ground black pepper

½ pound fresh snow peas, trimmed

1 large yellow (or red) bell pepper, cored, seeded, and
  sliced into ⅛-inch rounds

½ pound mushrooms, thinly sliced

1 Mix all the dressing ingredients in a covered jar and shake well.

2 Blanch the snow peas in boiling water for 1 minute.

3 Drain and refresh with cold running water. Pat dry with paper towels.

4 Combine the peas with the pepper and mushrooms; add enough dressing to coat.

Makes 6 cups

CHAPTER · 13

HEARTY SOUPS

Making a pot of soup is easy and can provide a solution for several dinners, and it's so convenient. With a little planning, these simple soups can be prepared in fifteen minutes, perhaps even tossed in a pot before going to work, so that they can be eaten with no further preparation when you arrive home. If you are beginning to get tired of your soup after the second or third time, be sure to freeze it instead of letting it get lost in the back of your refrigerator where it may spoil. You'll be glad you did when you come home late one night, only to be saved by those individual containers of your special blend.

 Corn Chowder with Potato Soup

Pureed Broccoli Soup

Pepper Pot Soup

Spinach Rice Soup

Cream of Spinach Soup

Chili

Chicken Noodle Soup

Split Pea Soup

Lentil Soup

CORN CHOWDER WITH POTATO SOUP

1 cup provides:
183 calories
81% carbohydrate
17% protein
2% fat
.5 g fat
2 mg cholesterol
0.1 g saturated fat
71 mg sodium
3.7 g fiber

3 cups fresh or frozen corn kernels, divided
1 tablespoon chopped onion
2½ cups nonfat or low-fat milk, divided
2 potatoes, baked, peeled, and diced
Freshly ground black pepper to taste

1 Puree 1 cup of the corn kernels, the onion, and 1 cup of the milk in a blender or food processor. Pour into a large saucepan.
2 Add the remaining 2 cups of corn kernels, remaining 1½ cups of milk, the potatoes and pepper and serve when heated through.

Makes 5 cups

PUREED BROCCOLI SOUP

1 cup provides:
142 calories
48% carbohydrate
29% protein
23% fat
4 g fat
13 mg cholesterol
2.3 g saturated fat
102 mg sodium
7.0 g fiber

1½ pounds broccoli, stemmed and chopped
3 cups low-fat milk
2 medium-size scallions, sliced
½ teaspoon salt
Freshly ground black pepper to taste

1 Combine all the ingredients in a medium saucepan.
2 Cover and cook over medium-low heat until the broccoli is tender, about 7 minutes.
3 Puree in a blender in batches until smooth.
4 Return the soup to the pan and warm through over medium-low heat. Serve.

NOTE: This soup is not only high in fiber, but also in vitamin C.

Makes 4 cups

PEPPER POT SOUP

1 cup provides:
102 calories
44% carbohydrate
33% protein
22% fat
2.5 g fat
18 mg cholesterol
0.6 g saturated fat
32 mg sodium
1.3 g fiber

1 teaspoon Puritan oil
4 ounces lean round steak or leftover steak
1 small onion, minced
2 stalks celery, finely chopped
2 green bell peppers, chopped
3½ cups water, divided
1 cup peeled and diced raw potatoes
2 tablespoons flour
½ teaspoon freshly ground black pepper
1 teaspoon dried marjoram
Salt to taste
½ cup low-fat plain yogurt

1 Place the oil in a pan, heat, and sauté the meat, onion, celery, and green peppers.
2 Add 3 cups of water and bring to a boil; add the potatoes, black pepper, marjoram, and salt, and simmer gently for 20 minutes, until the potatoes are tender.
3 Mix the flour with ⅓ cup of water and gradually blend into the soup.
4 Shortly before serving, reheat and add the yogurt.

Makes 5 cups

 # SPINACH RICE SOUP

1 cup provides:
77 calories
75% carbohydrate
23% protein
2% fat
.2 g fat
0.3 mg cholesterol
0.1 g saturated fat
73 mg sodium
1.3 g fiber

4–4½ cups chicken broth
1½ cups cooked rice
1 head fresh spinach, or 1 cup frozen spinach, thawed
Freshly ground pepper to taste
1 teaspoon finely grated Parmesan or Romano cheese

1 Combine 4 cups of chicken broth with the rice and spinach in a 2-quart saucepan over medium-high heat. Cook until heated through.
2 Season with pepper. Add more broth if a thinner consistency is desired. Heat to desired temperature.
3 Ladle into bowls. Garnish with cheese. Serve immediately.

Makes 6 cups

CREAM OF SPINACH SOUP

1 cup provides:
156 calories
74% carbohydrate
22% protein
4% fat
.7 g fat
1.9 mg cholesterol
0.2 g saturated fat
534 mg sodium
4.8 g fiber

1 10-ounce package frozen spinach
1 cup water
2 carrots, cut up
2 potatoes, quartered
1 onion, quartered
2⅓ cups nonfat or low-fat milk
⅓ cup flour
1 teaspoon salt
Freshly ground black pepper to taste
Pinch grated nutmeg

1 Steam the spinach in the water.
2 Steam the vegetables in water in a separate pan.
3 Puree the spinach and 1 cup of milk in a blender or food processor.
4 Add the other vegetables and puree.
5 Mix the flour and ⅓ cup of milk with a whisk or fork. Add the remaining 1 cup of milk and stir over low heat in a saucepan until thickened.
6 Add the vegetable mixture to the milk-flour mixture, and heat to desired temperature, about 2 to 3 minutes.
7 Add seasonings.

NOTE: This soup is high in fiber and vitamin A.

Makes 5 cups

CHILI

1 pound lean ground beef

1 medium onion, chopped

2 stalks celery, chopped

6 carrots, sliced

1 12-ounce can stewed tomatoes

2 12-ounce cans tomato sauce

1 12-ounce can pinto or kidney beans

3 teaspoons chili powder

Salt and pepper to taste

1 In a heavy skillet brown the beef, onion, and celery.
2 Add the remaining ingredients, and simmer until the carrots are tender, about 20 to 30 minutes.
3 Even better the next day.

NOTE: This soup is high in vitamin A and fiber.

Makes 8 cups

CHICKEN NOODLE SOUP

2 teaspoons Puritan oil

2 chicken breasts, skinned and cut into chunks

1 medium onion, chopped

¼ red bell pepper, chopped

1 tablespoon fresh rosemary, or ½ tablespoon dried

Salt and pepper

1 quart water

1 cup cooked noodles

3 carrots, sliced

2 stalks celery, finely chopped

1 Heat the oil in a heavy skillet and sauté the chicken breasts with the onion, celery, bell pepper, rosemary, and salt and pepper as needed.
2 Add the water and bring to a boil.
3 Add the noodles, carrots, and simmer until the carrots are tender, about 20 to 30 minutes.

Makes 6 cups

 # SPLIT PEA SOUP

1 cup provides:
190 calories
69% carbohydrate
28% protein
3% fat
.8 g fat
0 mg cholesterol
0 g saturated fat
11 mg sodium
1.1 g fiber

1 pound (2¼ cups) green split peas

2 quarts water

1 ham bone (the smallest one in the meat case)

1 small onion, chopped

Salt to taste

½ teaspoon black pepper

1 teaspoon dried marjoram

2 stalks celery, sliced

3 carrots, sliced or diced

1 Rinse the peas; in a pot combine the peas with the water, ham bone, onion, salt, pepper, and marjoram.
2 Bring to a boil, cover, reduce heat, and simmer (don't boil) for 1½ hours. *Note:* If using a Crockpot, proceed to this step, then continue when you get home. Stir occasionally.
3 Remove the bone and toss.
4 Add the celery and carrots and cook, uncovered, for 20 to 30 minutes, or until the vegetables are tender. (Or if you arrive home and want to eat soon, steam the carrots, then add to the soup and eat.)

OPTIONAL SEASONINGS: A few minutes before serving, add 2 tablespoons red wine, 1 teaspoon Dijon mustard, and ¼ teaspoon dried thyme.

Makes 10 cups

LENTIL SOUP

1 cup provides:
376 calories
68% carbohydrate
29% protein
3% fat
1 g fat
0 mg cholesterol
0.1 g saturated fat
467 mg sodium
1.9 g fiber

If you want beans and you don't have all day to cook, choose lentils, since they can be cooked tender in 20 minutes.

3 cups raw lentils, rinsed

1½ quarts water

1 teaspoon salt

1 clove garlic, crushed

1 onion, chopped

3 carrots, sliced

¼ teaspoon black pepper

1 12-ounce can whole tomatoes, chopped, with juice

2 tablespoons red wine

Juice of 1 lemon

1½ tablespoons molasses or brown sugar

1 tablespoon wine vinegar

1 Place the lentils, water, salt, garlic, onion, and carrots in a pot, and simmer, covered for 20 to 30 minutes.

2 Add the remaining ingredients, and simmer for another 15 to 20 minutes. (Soup is best made ahead, and enjoyed for several meals throughout the week.)

Makes 6 cups

CHAPTER · 14

MAIN DISHES

In the main-dish category, I have tried not to ignore the traditional American dinner of a piece of chicken, fish, or beef, accompanied by a vegetable or a salad and a bit of starch. But this way of eating is part of the problem with the American diet. It is restricting because animal protein portions should be limited to three to four ounces, and the serving sizes are always six to eight ounces minimum. Those who are watching weight or cholesterol are defeated before they start.

I use the protein as a seasoning with the rice, pasta, pizza crust, beans, or vegetables. This automatically cuts down the fat and cholesterol and increases the fiber. Calories are adjusted simply by increasing the ratio of vegetable to starch in the dish.

You'll find foods here that you grew up on, modified to meet the Fast-Food Diet criteria, while preserving the essence of your old favorites. They're all quick and easy to prepare.

Meats:

Barbecued (or Charred) Teriyaki Flank Steak

Shish Kabob with Lamb, Cherry Tomatoes, and Peppers

Turkey:

Roasted Turkey Breast

Turkey Burgers

Turkey Loaf with Carrots

Pizza:

Fresh Tomato Pizza

Mozzarella and Tomato Pizza with Spinach

Chicken:

Barbecued Chicken Breasts with Tabasco and Lime

Chicken Pot Roast with Rosemary and Garlic

Cajun Chicken

Rosemary Chicken with Artichoke Hearts

Chicken Enchiladas with Lettuce and Tomatoes

Coq au Vin

Chicken Parmesan with Pasta

Seafood:

Baked Swordfish Steaks with Lemon, Tomato and Cracked Peppercorns

Pan-Sautéed Snapper with Mushrooms and Bell Peppers

Blackened Halibut

Shrimp with Snow Peas

Shrimp with Garlic

Santa Fe Skewers with Shrimp

Scallops in Wine with Tomato

Pasta:

Spaghetti with Marinara Sauce

Spaghetti with Meat Sauce

Linguini with Clam Sauce

Pasta Primavera with Mushrooms, Peppers, and Broccoli

Pasta with Pesto Sauce

Fettucine with Mushrooms, Bell Peppers, and Peas in Lime Cream Sauce

Penne with Tomatoes, Capers, and Ricotta Cheese

Linguini with Shrimp and Broccoli

Fried Rice Combinations:

Fried Rice with Zucchini and Mushrooms

Spanish Fried Rice

Rice and Peas with Water Chestnuts

Tortilla Stuffers:

Fajitas with Chicken and Bell Peppers

Cuban-style Beef in Tortilla

Fish Taco with Cabbage

Although these would have been considered "side dishes" in my mother's kitchen, I find myself increasing the portion size and making a meal out of vegetables, perhaps along with a whole-grain roll or a slice of bread. In fact, I make it a point to eat at least one or two meatless dinners each week—no fish, chicken, or beef—and most of the time, no cheese—to cut back on saturated fat and cholesterol in my diet. Many who become accustomed to this type of meal actually prefer it and can understand why, even beyond the sixties' health-food fads, vegetarianism is not as farfetched an eating style as they once thought.

 Baked Potatoes Stuffed with Ricotta Cheese

Mashed Potatoes with Cabbage

Potato Fries

Zucchini-Carrot Stir-Fry

Zucchini with Onions, Tomatoes, and Basil

Steamed Carrots and Cauliflower with Dill

Green Bean Vinaigrette

Steamed Spaghetti Squash with Cracked Peppercorns

Spaghetti Squash with Marinara Sauce

BARBECUED (OR CHARRED) TERIYAKI
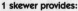 FLANK STEAK

4 ounces steak provides:
307 calories
5% carbohydrate
39% protein
56% fat
19 g fat
80 mg cholesterol
8 g saturated fat
1,008 mg sodium
0 g fiber

6 ounces steak provides:
451 calories
3% carbohydrate
40% protein
57% fat
28 g fat
120 mg cholesterol
12 g saturated fat
1,055 mg sodium
0 g fiber

MARINADE:

½ cup soy sauce

1 6-ounce can frozen concentrated pineapple juice

2 cloves garlic, crushed, or 1 teaspoon garlic powder

1 tablespoon fresh peeled ginger or ½ teaspoon powdered ginger

1 pound flank steak

1 Combine the marinade ingredients in a bowl.

2 Pour over the steak and let marinate for 1 or 2 hours, or overnight.

3 Broil or barbecue for 3 to 5 minutes on each side, depending on the thickness of the meat, for a rare steak.

NOTE: Compare the calorie and saturated fat difference from the two extra bites. Portion size is the key when choosing beef.

Makes 4 servings

SHISH KABOB WITH LAMB, CHERRY TOMATOES,
AND PEPPERS

1 skewer provides:
379 calories
14% carbohydrate
47% protein
39% fat
17 g fat
148 mg cholesterol
6.7 g saturated fat
118 mg sodium
4.5 g fiber

MARINADE:

1 cup lemon juice

1 tablespoon chopped onion

1 clove garlic, minced

1 tablespoon dried oregano

1 pound lamb, cut into cubes

12 pearl onions

12 medium-size mushrooms

12 cherry tomatoes

1 green bell pepper, cut into 2-inch squares

1 Combine all the marinade ingredients in a pan and stir well.

2 Marinate the lamb for 1 to 2 hours, or overnight.

3 Place all items on skewers, alternating meat, onion, mushroom, tomatoes and pepper.

4 Broil or barbecue, 10 to 12 minutes for medium rare, basting the entire skewer with marinade.

NOTE: Lamb is a higher fat meat, so the portion control provided by the shish kabob is helpful to keep fat intake in check.

Makes 4 servings

ROASTED TURKEY BREAST

3½ ounces breast provides:
175 calories
12% carbohydrate
82% protein
6% fat
1 g fat
94 mg cholesterol
0.4 g saturated fat
62 mg sodium
0 g fiber

3½ ounces dark meat with skin provides:
212 calories
0% carbohydrate
82% protein
36% fat
14 g fat
96 mg cholesterol
2.8 g saturated fat
89 mg sodium
0 g fiber

Juice of 1 lemon
1 turkey breast, skinned
Salt and pepper to taste
3 garlic cloves, crushed
2 teaspoons dried oregano

1 Squeeze the lemon juice directly onto the turkey breast.

2 Season with the salt and pepper, crushed garlic, and oregano.

3 Place the breast on a rack in a shallow pan and roast in a 425° oven for the first 15 minutes.

4 Reduce heat to 325° and roast, uncovered, for about 20 minutes per pound. Baste with lemon juice as desired.

NOTE: Both breast and dark meat are low in saturated fat.

TURKEY BURGERS

Serve on an onion roll with lettuce, tomato, onion, mustard, and catsup.

1 pound ground turkey
¼ cup finely chopped onion
2 tablespoons chopped green bell pepper
2 tablespoons chopped red bell pepper
Salt, pepper, garlic as desired

1 Mix all the ingredients together, and form into balls. (Due to the low fat content, the turkey has a tendency to fall apart. That is why the burgers begin as "balls" and end up being somewhat more similar to the classic burger.)
2 Barbecue or broil, turning when brown, 8 to 10 minutes or until any pink disappears inside.

NOTE: Ground turkey used in these recipes has 25 percent less fat than lean ground beef. This ground turkey is not as lean as white or dark meat of unground turkey because turkey skin is added to the meat during the grinding process.

NOTE: A 3½-ounce patty of cooked ground turkey contains 14 g fat while 3½ ounces lean ground beef contains 17 g fat. This is because the turkey skin is added to the meat.

Makes 4 burgers

 # TURKEY LOAF WITH CARROTS

1 whole egg
1 egg white
½ cup catsup, or 1 8-ounce can tomato sauce
¼ cup finely chopped onion
1 cup sliced carrots
½ teaspoon salt
1 teaspoon dried thyme

1 cup cooked rice, dried bread crumbs, or crushed
   cracker crumbs

1½ pounds ground turkey

1 Preheat the oven to 350°.

2 Combine all the ingredients in a mixing bowl and mix well.

3 Shape the mixture into a loaf and place in a 9"-×-5" baking dish.
Bake for about 1 hour.

Makes eight 3½-ounce servings

FRESH TOMATO PIZZA

Also known as pizza marinara, patrons in a true Italian restaurant are surprised to learn it is served with no cheese. Try it, you'll like it.

QUICK CRUSTS:

Split loaf of crusty French Bread

Split whole wheat pita bread

Boboli pizza crust

English muffin

Pillsbury instant pizza dough

(Some local pizza parlors sell dough separately, ready
   for you to bake)

NOT-SO-QUICK CRUST:

1¼ cups warm water

2 teaspoons yeast

1 tablespoon sugar

2 cups whole wheat flour

2 cups white flour

½ teaspoon salt

1 For a homemade crust, combine the first 3 ingredients and let
stand for 10 minutes.

2 Mix the flours and salt, then add the yeast mixture and knead for 10
to 15 minutes, or place in a food processor with a plastic bread blade
and process for 8 minutes.

(*continued on next page*)

TO ASSEMBLE:

Vegetable cooking spray

Cornmeal, if not using a nonstick pan

1 tablespoon olive oil

2 pounds plum tomatoes, peeled and sliced, or 1
    28-ounce can Italian plum tomatoes, well drained, and
    chopped

5 whole cloves garlic, thinly sliced

¼ cup chopped fresh basil or oregano leaves, or 2
    teaspoon dried

1 Preheat the oven to 450°. Choose the dough, and place it on a baking sheet that has been sprayed with vegetable cooking spray and dusted with cornmeal.

2 Brush the dough with the olive oil, then top with the tomatoes.

3 Sprinkle with the garlic and basil or oregano.

4 Bake the pizza for 10 minutes, or until the crust is brown and puffy. If using a quick crust follow these directions or toast the crust first, 3 minutes in the toaster oven or under the broiler, then add hot toppings. This is a particularly good idea for keeping the crust crispy when the toppings are moist.

Makes 6 servings

MOZZARELLA AND TOMATO PIZZA WITH SPINACH

1 serving provides:
282 calories
18% carbohydrate
34% protein
48% fat
6.5 g fat
105 mg cholesterol
5.6 g saturated fat
360 mg sodium
0.9 g fiber

If you insist that pizza isn't pizza without the cheese, try this recipe, with just the right amount of cheese to keep the pizza within the recommended guidelines for fat content.

1 Quick or Not-So-Quick Crust (see crust options from
    previous recipe)

Vegetable cooking spray

Cornmeal, if not using a nonstick pan

1 tablespoon olive oil

½ cup grated mozzarella or Romano cheese

Italian plum tomatoes, well drained, and chopped
1 cup chopped fresh spinach
¼ cup chopped fresh basil or oregano leaves, or 2
   teaspoons dried

1 Preheat the oven to 450°. Choose the dough, and place it on a baking sheet that has been sprayed with vegetable cooking spray and dusted with cornmeal. If using a quick crust, toast it first in toaster oven or broil to brown, 2 to 3 minutes.
2 Brush the dough with the olive oil, then top with the cheese, followed by the tomatoes and spinach.
3 Sprinkle with basil or oregano.
4 Bake for 10 minutes, or until the crust is brown and puffy. If using toasted quick crust, bake only till the cheese is melted.

Makes 6 servings

BARBECUED CHICKEN BREASTS WITH TABASCO AND LIME

1 skinless chicken breast half with marinade provides:
292 calories
4% carbohydrate
76% protein
20% fat
6 g fat
146 mg cholesterol
1.7 g saturated fat
170 mg sodium
0 g fiber

1 chicken breast half with barbecue sauce (traditional recipe) provides:
409 calories
4% carbohydrate
60% protein
36% fat
16 g fat
166 mg cholesterol
4.4 g saturated fat
392 mg sodium
0.3 g fiber

2 chicken breasts, halved, skinned
Juice of 1 lime
3 teaspoons Tabasco sauce
Freshly ground black pepper

1 Place the chicken breasts on a barbecue or broiler, alternately basting with the lime juice and Tabasco sauce.
2 Season with black pepper as desired.
3 Broil or barbecue for 5 minutes on each side, basting when turning, then an additional 5 minutes on each side, or till pink disappears and meat is still juicy.

Makes 4 servings

CHICKEN POT ROAST WITH ROSEMARY
AND GARLIC

1 chicken breast, 1 potato, and 1 carrot provide:
521 calories
39% carbohydrate
45% protein
16% fat
9.5 g fat
146 mg cholesterol
2.1 g saturated fat
167 mg sodium
6.4 g fiber

1 whole chicken, skinned or 4 whole chicken breasts, skinned

4 white potatoes

4 carrots, sliced

1 onion, quartered

1 tablespoon fresh rosemary, or 1 teaspoon dried

5 whole cloves garlic

2 teaspoons olive oil

1 Heat olive oil in heavy pan.

2 Place onion and garlic in hot oil and heat till onions are translucent.

3 Add remaining vegetables, sprinkle with rosemary and bake at 425° for 10 minutes, then cover and reduce heat to 350° and bake for an additional 35 minutes.

4 Add water as needed, up to 1 cup.

Makes 4 servings

CAJUN CHICKEN

1 chicken breast half provides:
284 calories
0% carbohydrate
79% protein
21% fat
6 g fat
146 mg cholesterol
1.7 g saturated fat
126 mg sodium
0 g fiber

2 chicken breasts, halved, skinned

Cajun seasonings

1 Place the chicken breasts on a barbecue or broiler.

2 Season with the Cajun spices as desired, and cook for a total of 10 to 12 minutes on each side, turning twice.

NOTE: You'll find Cajun seasonings in the spice section of your supermarket, or at the fish or meat market counter.

Makes 4 servings

ROSEMARY CHICKEN WITH ARTICHOKE HEARTS

1 chicken breast and 1 sourdough slice provide:
325 calories
12% carbohydrate
69% protein
19% fat
6.5 g fat
146 mg cholesterol
1.7 g saturated fat
146 mg sodium
0.6 g fiber

1 whole chicken, or 4 chicken breasts, skinned
1 onion, quartered
1 tablespoon fresh rosemary, or 2 teaspoons dried
5 whole cloves garlic
1 4-ounce jar artichoke hearts, half drained
4 slices sourdough bread

1 Place all the ingredients in a heavy pan and bake at 425° for 10 minutes, then cover and reduce heat to 350° and bake for an additional 35 minutes.
2 Serve with hot sourdough bread, unbuttered.

Makes 4 servings

CHICKEN ENCHILADAS WITH LETTUCE AND TOMATOES

1 enchilada with topping provides:
345 calories
30% carbohydrate
49% protein
21% fat
8 g fat
100 mg cholesterol
1.7 g saturated fat
655 mg sodium
2.7 g fiber

3 cups store-bought enchilada sauce
4 skinless chicken breasts, cooked
6 corn tortillas
1 ounce mozzarella cheese, grated
2 cups shredded lettuce
2 cups chopped fresh tomatoes
4 ounces nonfat or low-fat plain yogurt

1 Preheat the oven to 375°. Place 1 cup of the enchilada sauce in a shallow baking dish.
2 Cut up the chicken breasts and place in the tortillas, folding the edges over, and placing in the baking dish.
3 Top with the remaining enchilada sauce, and bake for 25 minutes, or until heated through.
4 Remove from the oven and top with the cheese, lettuce, tomatoes, and yogurt

Makes 6 servings.

COQ AU VIN

1 chicken breast half provides:
344 calories
9% carbohydrate
66% protein
22% fat
8.5 g fat
146 mg cholesterol
2.0 g saturated fat
313 mg sodium
1.7 g fiber

1 teaspoon Puritan oil

3 chicken breasts, halved, skinned

1 medium onion, chopped

1 clove garlic, crushed

16 whole mushrooms

2 cups dry red wine

1⅓ cups beef stock, canned, such as Swanson's, with fat skimmed from top

2 tablespoons flour

1 tablespoon dried thyme

1 Heat the oil in a large skillet and brown the chicken with the onion, garlic, and mushrooms.

2 Add the wine, 1 cup of beef stock, and thyme, bring to a boil, and simmer for 20 minutes.

3 Mix the flour with ⅓ cup of beef stock and slowly add to the chicken sauce, heating until the sauce thickens, about 1½ minutes.

4 Serve with French bread.

NOTE: Keep canned beef broth in the refrigerator, to harden fat for easy removal.

Makes 6 servings

CHICKEN PARMESAN WITH PASTA

1 chicken breast half, ¼ cup sauce, and ½ cup pasta provide:
640 calories
35% carbohydrate
43% protein
19% fat
13.5 g fat
155 mg cholesterol
4.9 g saturated fat
379 mg sodium
1.7 g fiber

1 onion, chopped

2 chicken breasts, halved, skinned

1 cup (store-bought) spaghetti sauce

½ cup white wine

¼ cup grated Parmesan cheese

2 cups cooked pasta

1 Using a large nonstick skillet, sauté the onion and chicken, browning on each side.

2 Stir in the marinara sauce and wine and allow to simmer, uncovered, until cooked, about 20 minutes.

3 Before serving, add the Parmesan cheese.

4 Serve over the pasta of your choice.

NOTE: See page 217 for ratings of bottled spaghetti sauce.

Makes 4 servings

BAKED SWORDFISH STEAKS WITH LEMON, TOMATO, AND CRACKED PEPPERCORNS

3 ounces fish and ½ tomato provide:
160 calories
7% carbohydrate
63% protein
30% fat
5 g fat
43 mg cholesterol
1.2 g saturated fat
98 mg sodium
1.0 g fiber

6 ounces fish and ½ tomato provide:
320 calories
7% carbohydrate
63% protein
30% fat
10.5 g fat
86 mg cholesterol
2.4 g saturated fat
196 mg sodium
1.0 g fiber

4 4-ounce swordfish steaks, rinsed and patted dry
1 teaspoon olive oil
Fresh parsley or cilantro, chopped (optional)
2 tomatoes, sliced
2 lemons, 1 sliced, other halved
Black peppercorns cracked, to taste

1 Preheat the oven to 425°. Place aluminum foil (large enough to completely wrap fish) on a baking pan, and place steaks on the foil.

2 Brush the steaks with the olive oil, followed by the juice of 1 lemon.

3 Season with the cracked black peppercorns, then arrange the tomato slices and lemon slices alternately on top. Sprinkle with fresh parsley or cilantro, if desired.

4 Wrap the fish with the foil, and bake for 10 to 15 minutes (10 minutes per inch of thickness of fish).

Makes 4 servings

PAN-SAUTÉED SNAPPER WITH MUSHROOMS AND BELL PEPPERS

3 ounces fish and ½ pepper provide:
144 calories
12% carbohydrate
68% protein
19% fat
3 g fat
41 mg cholesterol
0.5 g saturated fat
73 mg sodium
1.3 g fiber

6 ounces fish and ½ pepper provide:
288 calories
12% carbohydrate
68% protein
19% fat
6 g fat
82 mg cholesterol
0.5 g saturated fat
146 mg sodium
2.6 g fiber

1 teaspoon Puritan oil
16 mushrooms, sliced
1 green bell pepper, diced
1 red bell pepper, diced
1 pound red snapper or orange roughy
Juice of 1 lemon
Salt and pepper

1 Place the oil in a hot skillet, add the mushrooms and peppers, and sauté until peppers have softened.
2 Add the fish, and cook at high temperature for 2 to 3 minutes on each side.
3 Add the lemon juice and season as desired with salt and pepper.

Makes 4 servings

BLACKENED HALIBUT

4 ounces fish provides:
217 calories
1% carbohydrate
55% protein
45% fat
11 g fat
68 mg cholesterol
0.4 g saturated fat
152 mg sodium
0 g fiber

2 teaspoons Puritan oil
1 pound halibut
Cajun seasonings

1 Heat the oil in a heavy skillet.
2 Place the fish in the oil, seasoning with the Cajun spices.
3 Cook for 5 minutes on each side.

NOTE: Cajun seasonings are a blend of spices often containing salt, red pepper, chili peppers, garlic, et cetera, and can generally be found with other seasonings in the supermarket or at the meat or fish counter.

Makes 4 servings

SHRIMP WITH SNOW PEAS

3 ounces shrimp with ½
cup snow peas and 1
cup steamed rice
provides:
389 calories
64% carbohydrate
30% protein
5% fat
2.5 g fat
170 mg cholesterol
0.2 g saturated fat
172 mg sodium
8.3 g fiber

1 teaspoon Puritan oil

1 clove garlic, crushed

1 pound snow peas, trimmed, strings removed

16 medium-size fresh shrimp, cleaned and deveined

1 tablespoon white wine

4 cups steamed rice

1 Heat the oil in a heavy skillet.
2 Add the garlic and heat for 1 minute.
3 Add the snow peas and shrimp, and toss for 2 minutes.
4 Add the wine and heat for 1 additional minute.
5 Serve with the rice.

Makes 4 servings

SHRIMP WITH GARLIC

4 shrimp provide:
172 calories
9% carbohydrate
27% protein
5% fat
5 g fat
224 mg cholesterol
2.5 g saturated fat
242 mg sodium
0.2 g fiber

2 teaspoons butter or margarine

1 scallion, minced

3 cloves garlic, minced

16 medium-size shrimp, shelled and deveined

Lemon wedges

2 tablespoons finely chopped parsley

1 Melt the butter in a nonstick skillet.
2 Stir in the scallion and garlic; cook until soft.
3 Add the shrimp and cook until the pink disappears, 3 to 5 minutes.
4 Squeeze the lemon over each serving. Sprinkle with the parsley.
5 Serve with stir-fried vegetables and rice.

Makes 2 servings

SANTA FE SKEWERS WITH SHRIMP

1 skewer provides:
150 calories
33% carbohydrate
59% protein
8% fat
1.5 g fat
170 mg cholesterol
0.1 g saturated fat
168 mg sodium
2.8 g fiber

MARINADE:

1 cup lemon juice

1 tablespoon chopped onion

1 clove garlic, minced

1 tablespoon fresh cilantro or dried coriander

1 pound shrimp, cleaned, deveined

12 pearl onions

12 medium-size mushrooms

12 cherry tomatoes

1 green bell pepper, cut into 2-inch squares

1 Combine all the marinade ingredients in a pan and stir well.
2 Marinate the shrimp in it for 1 hour.
3 Place all items on 4 skewers, alternating shrimp, onion, mushroom, tomato, and pepper.
4 Broil or barbecue 5 to 10 minutes, turning frequently and basting each entire skewer with the marinade.

Makes 4 servings

SCALLOPS IN WINE WITH TOMATO

4 ounces scallops provide:
182 calories
12% carbohydrate
58% protein
25% fat
5 g fat
60 mg cholesterol
0.4 g saturated fat
314 mg sodium
1 g fiber

1 tablespoon olive oil

1 pound fresh or frozen scallops, rinsed and patted dry

¼ cup dry white wine

2 tomatoes, chopped

2 tablespoons fresh basil, or 1 teaspoon dried

Freshly ground black pepper to taste

1 Heat the olive oil in a skillet and brown the scallops at a high temperature for 1 minute.
2 Add the wine, tomatoes, and basil. Season with black pepper.

Makes 4 servings

SPAGHETTI WITH MARINARA SAUCE

1 cup pasta with ½ cup sauce provides:
214 calories
68% carbohydrate
14% protein
18% fat
4 g fat
0 mg cholesterol
0.5 g saturated fat
372 mg sodium
2.0 g fiber

½ cup Bottled Spaghetti Sauce provides:
136 calories
56% carbohydrate
6% protein
38% fat
6 g fat
0 mg cholesterol
0.8 g saturated fat
618 mg sodium
1.0 g fiber

½ cup our marinara sauce provides:
60 calories
37% carbohydrate
15% protein
46% fat
3 g fat
0 mg cholesterol
0.4 g saturated fat
371 mg sodium
1 g fiber

1 pound fresh spaghetti or 1 package dry spaghetti noodles

MARINARA SAUCE:

1 tablespoon olive oil

1 clove garlic, minced

2½ cups canned or fresh tomatoes (try Progresso crushed puree with bits)

6 finely chopped anchovies

½ teaspoon dried oregano

1 tablespoon chopped fresh parsley

2 cups cooked spaghetti

1 Add spaghetti to a large pan of boiling water, cooking until tender (8 to 10 minutes for dry, 3 to 5 minutes for fresh). Drain.
2 In a heavy skillet heat the olive oil and sauté the garlic.
3 Add the tomatoes, anchovies, oregano, and parsley.
4 Bring to a boil, then reduce heat and simmer, uncovered, for 15 minutes, stirring occasionally.
5 Serve over spaghetti.

NOTE: There are many types of pasta available in stores today. Fresh pasta in the deli packages of 8 to 9 ounces cook to double that weight, and you have about 4 cups. This is more than you would get from an 8-ounce package of dry pasta. That's why pasta is listed as cups in the ingredients.

VARIATION: Add sliced zucchini and whole mushrooms along with the tomatoes to increase the vegetables.

NOTE: If you use bottled spaghetti sauce, simply dilute 2 cups sauce with ⅓ cup white wine, and add zucchini and mushrooms.

Makes 4 servings; 2 cups sauce

SPAGHETTI WITH MEAT SAUCE

½ cup pasta with ½ cup sauce provides:
344 calories
52% carbohydrate
22% protein
26% fat
10 g fat
35 mg cholesterol
3.5 g saturated fat
31 mg sodium
1.8 g fiber

Many people already have their own favorite recipe for making old-fashioned spaghetti sauce. The purpose of this recipe is to add meat in proportion that will keep the dish at an acceptably low level of fat and cholesterol, while still presenting a tasty familiar dish.

1 pound fresh spaghetti noodles or 1 package dry
  spaghetti noodles

MEAT SAUCE
1 recipe Marinara Sauce (see above) or 2 cups spaghetti
  sauce
½ pound extra-lean ground beef
1 pound mushrooms, sliced
1 zucchini, sliced

1 Add spaghetti to a large pot of boiling water, cooking until tender (8 to 10 minutes for dry pasta and 3 to 5 minutes for fresh). Drain.
2 Brown the ground beef in a heavy skillet without adding additional fat.
3 Add the mushrooms and zucchini and brown for 1 minute.
4 Add the marinara sauce and simmer for 10 minutes.
5 Serve sauce over pasta.

Makes 4 servings; 2 cups sauce

 # LINGUINI WITH CLAM SAUCE

1 cup pasta with ½ cup sauce provides:
220 calories
61% carbohydrate
17% protein
22% fat
5 g fat
30 mg cholesterol
0.8 g saturated fat
561 mg sodium
1.1 g fiber

1 pound dry linguini
1 tablespoon olive oil
2 cloves garlic, minced
6½ ounces clams, heated, undrained
¼ cup finely chopped fresh parsley
1 tablespoon grated Parmesan or Romano cheese

1 Cook the noodles until al dente; drain.
2 In a skillet heat the olive oil and sauté the garlic.
3 Add the clams, and heat for 30 seconds.
4 Toss the pasta, parsley, and cheese with the clam sauce.

Makes 4 to 6 servings, or 5 cups pasta.

PASTA PRIMAVERA WITH MUSHROOMS, PEPPERS, AND BROCCOLI

1 cup pasta with ½ cup sauce provides:
172 calories
58% carbohydrate
23% protein
19% fat
3.5 g fat
31 mg cholesterol
1.6 g saturated fat
174 mg sodium
4.3 g fiber

1 pound fresh spaghetti or 1 1-pound package dry vermicelli noodles
3 cups broccoli florets or other fresh vegetables
2 cups mushrooms, whole
1 tablespoon cornstarch
1 cup chicken stock
1 cup grated Parmesan cheese
1 red bell pepper or small tomato, diced

1 Add the spaghetti to a large pan of boiling water, cooking until tender (8 to 10 minutes for dry, 3 to 5 minutes for fresh). Drain.
2 Steam the broccoli or other vegetables until crisp-tender.
3 In a saucepan over medium heat, combine the cornstarch with ¼ cup of chicken stock; mix until the cornstarch dissolves.
4 Add the remaining ¾ cup of stock and bring to a boil.
5 Reduce the heat, stirring constantly until thickened.
6 Toss the broccoli, pasta, sauce, and Parmesan cheese, combining thoroughly.
7 Garnish with the diced tomato or pepper.

NOTE: ½ pound dry spaghetti noodles cooks up to 2½ cups of pasta.

Makes 4 to 6 servings

PASTA WITH PESTO SAUCE

1 cup pasta with 1 tablespoon pesto sauce provides:

218 calories
58% carbohydrate
10% protein
33% fat
8 g fat
0.6 mg cholesterol
1 g saturated fat
16 mg sodium
1 g fiber

Since this sauce is more work than the typical fast fooder may engage in, we suggest that you get a little help from the fresh pesto sauce in your supermarket deli or even a specialty Italian deli.

1 pound dry pasta
¼ cup olive oil
1 tablespoon grated Parmesan cheese
½ cup chopped fresh basil or 2 ounces bottled pesto sauce
or
1 tablespoon prepared pesto sauce
1 cup pasta

1 Add pasta to a large pot of boiling water, cooking until tender (8 to 10 minutes). Drain.
2 Add oil, cheese, and basil to pasta and toss. If using the prepared pesto sauce, stir the sauce, and add 1 tablespoon per cup of pasta. Toss well and serve immediately.

Makes 4 to 6 servings, or 5 cups pasta.

FETTUCINE WITH MUSHROOMS, BELL PEPPERS, AND PEAS IN LIME CREAM SAUCE

1 cup pasta with sauce provides:

144 calories
68% carbohydrate
20% protein
12% fat
2 g fat
4 mg cholesterol
0.9 g saturated fat
113 mg sodium
2.7 g fiber

3 cups snow peas, chopped red and green bell peppers and sliced mushrooms
1 tablespoon cornstarch
1 cup nonfat or low-fat milk
½ cup frozen peas
Juice of 1 lime, or 3 tablespoons lime juice
4 cups cooked fettucine
¼ cup grated Parmesan cheese

1 Steam the vegetables until crisp-tender, set aside.

2 In a saucepan over medium heat, combine the cornstarch with ¼ cup of milk; mix until the cornstarch dissolves.

3 Add the remaining ¾ cup of milk and bring to a boil.

4 Reduce the heat, add the peas, and stir constantly until thickened.

5 Add the lime juice and stir.

6 Toss the vegetables, pasta, sauce, and Parmesan cheese, combining thoroughly.

Makes 4 to 6 servings

PENNE WITH TOMATOES, CAPERS, AND RICOTTA CHEESE

1 cup pasta with ½ cup sauce provides:
293 calories
59% carbohydrate
16% protein
25% fat
60 mg cholesterol
2.0 g saturated fat
474 mg sodium
2.9 g fiber

1 tablespoon olive oil

1 small onion, chopped

2 tomatoes, chopped

½ cup part-skim ricotta cheese

4 cups cooked penne (tube-shape pasta) or any other pasta

2 tablespoons capers

1 tablespoon chopped fresh parsley

1 Heat the olive oil in a skillet and sauté the onion.

2 Add the tomatoes and heat for 2 minutes.

3 Add the ricotta cheese, if desired, and stir well.

4 Toss the pasta, capers, and parsley with the sauce.

Makes 4 to 6 servings

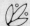 # LINGUINI WITH SHRIMP AND BROCCOLI

1 cup pasta, 2 ounces shrimp, and ½ cup broccoli provide:
200 calories
24% carbohydrate
36% protein
16% fat
3.5 g fat
113 mg cholesterol
0.3 g saturated fat
111 mg sodium
1.8 g fiber

1 bunch broccoli, florets only, approximately 2 cups
1 tablespoon olive oil
2 cloves garlic, minced
¾ pound shrimp, shelled and deveined
4 cups cooked linguini
¼ cup finely chopped fresh parsley

1 Steam the broccoli.
2 Heat the olive oil in a skillet and sauté the garlic.
3 Add the shrimp and sauté for 3 minutes, until lightly browned, not overcooked.
4 Toss the pasta, parsley, and broccoli with the shrimp.

Makes 4 to 6 servings

 # FRIED RICE WITH ZUCCHINI AND MUSHROOMS

1 cup provides:
77 calories
76% carbohydrate
9% protein
15% fat
1 g fat
0 mg cholesterol
0.2 g saturated fat
11 mg sodium
1.4 g fiber

1 teaspoon Puritan oil
1 zucchini, sliced
1 cup sliced mushrooms
1 stalk celery, sliced
1 cup leftover cooked rice, chilled
Low-sodium soy sauce (optional)

1 Heat the oil in a heavy skillet. Add all the vegetables and soy sauce, if desired; stir over high heat.
2 Toss in the rice; heat thoroughly.

Makes 4 cups

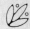 # SPANISH FRIED RICE

1 cup provides:
101 calories
77% carbohydrate
10% protein
13% fat
1.5 g fat
0 mg cholesterol
0.2 g saturated fat
336 mg sodium
1.8 g fiber

1 teaspoon Puritan oil
3 scallions, chopped
1 green bell pepper, chopped
1 can diced green chilies
1 1-pound can tomatoes, drained and diced
1 tablespoon Worcestershire sauce
¼ teaspoon black pepper
1 cup leftover cooked rice, chilled

1 Heat the oil in a heavy skillet, add the vegetables and seasonings, and stir over high heat.
2 Toss in the rice; heat thoroughly.

Makes 4 cups

 # RICE AND PEAS WITH WATER CHESTNUTS

1 cup provides:
111 calories
79% carbohydrate
11% protein
10% fat
1 g fat
0 mg cholesterol
0.2 g saturated fat
313 mg sodium
2.7 g fiber

1 teaspoon Puritan oil
¾ cup frozen peas
1 4-ounce can water chestnuts
1 tablespoon coarse-ground garlic powder
¼ teaspoon black pepper
1 cup leftover cooked rice, chilled

1 Heat the oil in a heavy skillet, add the vegetables and seasonings, and stir over high heat.
2 Toss in the rice; heat thoroughly

Makes 4 cups

FAJITAS WITH CHICKEN AND BELL PEPPERS

1 tortilla serving provides:

263 calories
33% carbohydrate
46% protein
22% fat
6.5 g fat
72 mg cholesterol
1.0 g saturated fat
64 mg sodium
0.8 g fiber

This popular Mexican dish has been traditionally made with beef, but has become a catchall term for make-it-yourself burritos filled with grilled chicken, fish, *or* beef.

1 teaspoon Puritan oil or other unflavored oil
2 cloves garlic
1 large onion, cut into bite-size chunks
2 bell peppers, cut into strips
4 chicken breasts, cut into bite-size pieces (may substitute lean beef such as flank steak, or a firm white fish, such as halibut or shark).
1 teaspoon ground cumin
1 teaspoon dried oregano
Black pepper to taste
½ cup lime juice
4 flour tortillas
Salsa
Chopped scallions

1 Heat the oil in a skillet and add the garlic, onion, peppers, and chicken, browning for about 2 minutes.
2 Add the seasonings and lime juice and simmer until done, about 7 more minutes.
3 Warm the tortillas in a nonstick pan, turning as needed with tongs, just until softened (15 to 30 seconds). Top with the chicken mixture. Fold up the bottom, then fold in the sides to enclose.
4 Garnish with salsa and scallions, if desired.

Makes 4 servings

CUBAN-STYLE BEEF IN TORTILLA

1 medium onion, diced

1 clove garlic, minced

1 green bell pepper, diced

1 pound lean ground beef, or 1 pound ground turkey

⅛ teaspoon black pepper

1 tablespoon chopped capers or green olives

2 tablespoons raisins

1 potato, cooked or baked, and chilled (optional)

8 flour tortillas, heated

1 recipe Spanish Fried Rice (page 223)

1 Using a nonstick skillet, sauté the onion, garlic, and pepper until translucent.

2 Add the beef and pepper and cook until the meat is browned.

3 Drain any fat from the meat and add the capers and raisins, and, if you choose, the diced potato.

4 Spoon the filling into the hot tortillas, roll up, and serve with the rice.

NOTE: Since the beef in a tortilla is 40 percent fat, adding ½ cup Spanish rice gives a better nutritional effect.

Makes 8 servings

FISH TACO WITH CABBAGE

1 Fish Taco with 1 tablespoon plain, low-fat yogurt provides:
184 calories
33% carbohydrate
42% protein
25% fat
5 g fat
30 mg cholesterol
0.1 g saturated fat
118 mg sodium
1.6 g fiber

1 breaded and fried fish taco with avocado and sour cream in fried tortilla provides:
319 calories
21% carbohydrate
18% protein
61% fat
21.5 g fat
35 mg cholesterol
3.6 g saturated fat
104 mg sodium
2.3 g fiber

2 tablespoons lemon juice
Dash of chili powder
2 tablespoons chopped fresh cilantro
1 14½-ounce can chicken broth
½ pound red snapper or other firm white-fleshed fish
    fillet or fish leftover from last night's dinner
4 corn tortillas
Garnish of your choice: shredded cabbage, cilantro,
    yogurt, salsa, tomato

1 In a nonstick pan, bring the lemon juice, chile, cilantro, and broth to a boil.
2 Add the fish fillets and simmer for 7 to 10 minutes, until the fish flakes when tested with a fork. Drain.
3 While the fish is cooking, warm the tortillas in a microwave or in a nonstick pan.
4 Place in each tortilla 2 ounces of fish and the garnishes.

NOTE: Make fish tacos from last night's dinner. Simply reheat the fish in the microwave for 1½ minutes or in a nonstick pan using vegetable cooking spray. Fill tortillas and garnish.

Makes 4 servings

BAKED POTATOES STUFFED WITH RICOTTA CHEESE

1 stuffed baked potato provides:
248 calories
59% carbohydrate
16% protein
25% fat
7 g fat
19 mg cholesterol
3–4 g saturated fat
106 mg sodium
3.8 g fiber

2 medium potatoes
1 teaspoon margarine
3 scallions, chopped
½ cup part-skim ricotta cheese

1 Preheat oven to 400°
2 Bake the potatoes for 1 hour in a 400° oven, or for 10 minutes in a microwave oven.

3 When slightly cooled, split the tops and remove the pulp, reserving the shells.

4 Heat the margarine in a skillet and sauté the scallions.

5 Add the pulp and ricotta cheese; heat until thoroughly warm.

6 Stuff the potato shells with the ricotta mixture and serve.

Makes 2 servings

 # MASHED POTATOES WITH CABBAGE

1 cup provides:
165 calories
75% carbohydrate
10% protein
15% fat
3 g fat
3 mg cholesterol
0.9 g saturated fat
57 mg sodium
2.6 g fiber

Both the Irish and the Scots claim this concoction as "native fare," each calling it *colcannon*, which translates as cabbage or white-headed kale. I have lowered the fat to make it a perfect balance of nutrients.

4 cups thinly sliced green cabbage

6 boiling potatoes, peeled and quartered

1 tablespoon butter or margarine

6 scallions, including 2" of top, cut into ⅛" slices

1 cup low-fat milk

Salt and pepper

1 Steam both the cabbage and potatoes for 10 minutes, or until tender.

2 Melt the butter or margarine in a skillet and add the scallions, then add the cabbage.

3 Mash the potatoes with the milk, using an electric mixer or food processor.

4 Add the potatoes to the cabbage and season to your liking.

Makes 6 cups

POTATO FRIES

5-ounce potato provides:
153 calories
86% carbohydrate
8% protein
6% fat
1 g fat
0 mg cholesterol
0.2 g saturated fat
19 mg sodium
3.7 g fiber

French fries, same weight as medium baked potato, provides:
505 calories
47% carbohydrate
5% protein
47% fat
26 g fat
21 mg cholesterol
0 g saturated fat
250 mg sodium
0 g fiber

4 leftover medium baked potatoes, chilled
1 teaspoon margarine

1 Slice the potatoes into strips, like large French fries.
2 Melt the margarine in a nonstick pan over high heat and sauté the potatoes until brown.
3 Serve with catsup if desired.

Makes 4 1-cup servings, depending on size of potatoes

NOTE: Nutritional analysis compares equal weight, 5.5 ounces, for baked potato and fries. A large serving of fries at a typical fast-food restaurant weighs about 4 ounces. Obviously restaurant servings vary.

ZUCCHINI-CARROT STIR-FRY

1 serving provides:
65 calories
57% carbohydrate
10% protein
33% fat
2.5 g fat
0 mg cholesterol
0.3 g saturated fat
26 mg sodium
3.3 g fiber

2 carrots
1 zucchini
1 teaspoon olive oil
1 tablespoon chopped fresh basil (or omit oil and basil and add 2 teaspoons pesto sauce)

1 Cut the carrots and zucchini into match stick–size julienne.
2 Heat the oil in a skillet, and toss the carrots and zucchini in the hot oil for 3 minutes, or until crisp-tender.
3 Add the basil and toss just before serving.

Makes 2 servings

ZUCCHINI WITH ONIONS, TOMATOES, AND BASIL

1 cup vegetables plus 1 cup rice provides:
271 calories
83% carbohydrate
8% protein
9% fat
2.5 g fat
0 mg cholesterol
0.3 g saturated fat
96 mg sodium
3.5 g fiber

2 teaspoons olive oil
1 small onion, chopped
1 green bell pepper, cut into chunks
1 medium zucchini, cut into ¼" slices
1 7½-ounce can tomatoes, cut up
⅛ teaspoon dried oregano or basil
1 tablespoon white wine or sherry
4 cups cooked rice

1 In a nonstick pan heat the olive oil, sauté the onion until tender over low heat.
2 Add the green pepper, zucchini, undrained tomatoes, oregano or basil, and wine.
3 Bring to a boil, reduce heat and simmer, uncovered, for 5 to 10 minutes, or until the vegetables are tender. (Tastes great reheated.)
4 Serve over the rice.

Makes 4 cups

STEAMED CARROTS AND CAULIFLOWER WITH DILL

1 cup provides:
45 calories
64% carbohydrate
13% protein
24% fat
1 g fat
0 mg cholesterol
0.2 g saturated fat
26 mg sodium
2.9 g fiber

1 head cauliflower, cut into bite-size pieces
3 carrots, sliced
1 teaspoon olive oil
½ teaspoon dried dill

1 Place the vegetables in a steamer basket, in a pot of boiling water. Steam for 5 minutes, or until the vegetables are tender.
2 Drizzle the olive oil onto the vegetables and sprinkle with dill.

Makes 4 cups

GREEN BEAN VINAIGRETTE

4 ounces beans with 2 teaspoons marinade provides:
61 calories
53% carbohydrate
13% protein
34% fat
2.5 g fat
0 mg cholesterol
0.4 g saturated fat
20 mg sodium
2.1 g fiber

VINAIGRETTE:

1 tablespoon white wine vinegar

2 teaspoons Puritan oil

1 teaspoon Dijon mustard

Salt and pepper to taste

1 pound green beans, washed and trimmed

1 Mix the ingredients for the vinaigrette.
2 Steam the green beans for 4 minutes, or until tender.
3 Toss the beans with the vinaigrette. Serve hot or cold.

Makes 4 servings

STEAMED SPAGHETTI SQUASH WITH CRACKED PEPPERCORNS

1 cup squash provides:
62 calories
62% carbohydrate
6% protein
32% fat
4.5 g fat
0 mg cholesterol
0.4 g saturated fat
50 mg sodium
2.2 g fiber

1 spaghetti squash, halved and seeded

1 teaspoon margarine

Salt to taste

Peppercorns, cracked, to taste

1 Steam the squash for 20 minutes, or until tender.
2 With a fork, dig out the meat of the squash, which appears as spaghetti.
3 Season with the margarine, salt, and fresh cracked peppercorns, and serve as a side dish or main dish along with a salad and whole-grain roll.

Number of servings varies with size of squash, from 4 to 6 cups

SPAGHETTI SQUASH WITH MARINARA SAUCE

2 cups squash, ⅓ cup sauce, ¼ cup Parmesan, roll, salad, and 1 teaspoon dressing provide:

373 calories
52% carbohydrate
17% protein
31% fat
13 g fat
15 mg cholesterol
4.2 g saturated fat
980 mg sodium
3.7 g fiber

1 spaghetti squash, halved and seeded

1 cup marinara sauce (bottled or see recipe, page 217)

¾ cup grated Parmesan cheese

1 Steam the squash for 20 minutes, or until tender.

2 Meanwhile, heat the marinara sauce in a saucepan.

3 With a fork, dig out the meat of the squash, which appears as spaghetti.

4 Pour the hot marinara sauce over the squash and toss with the cheese.

5 Serve as a side dish or main dish along with a salad and a whole-grain roll.

NOTE: This recipe is high in sodium due to the Parmesan cheese.

Number of servings varies with size of squash, from 4 to 6 cups

CHAPTER · 15

PARTY SNACKS

If you live fast and like action, chances are you enjoy parties. Having friends in your home for drinks and snacks can be fun and easy if you mix a few carry-out items along with some treats you have put together yourself. These gatherings generally turn into dinners, without formally being called dinners, and the casual nature makes it lots of fun for everyone after long, hard days of work. There's nothing wrong with snacks for dinner, as long as they abide by our nutritional principles.

Begin by selecting a theme. I have listed four themes for a last-minute party: Oriental, Mexican, Italian, and Greek. Each one includes a vegetable platter and dip or marinade relating to the cuisine. The ingredients, from egg rolls to tortilla chips, from garlic toasts to pasta salad, can either be purchased at a deli or restaurant, or prepared according to my simple recipes. When your friends arrive, you can light the candles, sit down, relax, and enjoy.

 Oriental:

Vegetable Platter: Chinese peas, cauliflower, scallions, and red bell pepper

Fresh Pineapple

Ginger Marinade

Potstickers

Mexican:

Spicy Yogurt Dip

Quesadilla with Cheese and Cilantro

Baked Tortilla Chips

Mexican Bean Dip

Kitchen Sink Nachos with Bean, Cheese, and Salsa

Pineapple Salsa

Italian:

Eggplant Slices with Marinara and Parmesan

Antipasto with Vinaigrette

Mushrooms in Sherry and Tarragon

Roman Grilled Garlic Toast with Roma Tomatoes

Greek:

Cucumber Yogurt Dip

Cajun Pita Triangles

 # GINGER MARINADE

1 tablespoon provides:
25 calories
32% carbohydrate
9% protein
1% fat
0 g fat
1 mg cholesterol
0 g saturated fat
258 mg sodium
0.1 g fiber

2 tablespoons dry sherry

3 slices fresh ginger

4 scallions

1 tablespoon oyster sauce

1 Crush the sherry, ginger, and scallions in a blender.

2 Strain the mixture, and mix it with the oyster sauce.

3 Serve as a dip with egg rolls or fresh vegetables.

Makes ¼ cup

POTSTICKERS

FILLING:

½ pound ground turkey

1 cup minced cabbage

2 scallions, minced

1 egg, or 2 egg whites

1 tablespoon light soy sauce

½ teaspoon grated orange peel

½ teaspoon chili oil (optional)

1 teaspoon Puritan oil

40 won ton skins, 2" × 2" square, cut into largest circle possible
Cornstarch for dusting
Oil
1 cup water

1 Combine the filling ingredients in a large bowl and mix well.

2 Set 1 rounded teaspoon of filling in the center of each won ton skin.

3 Moisten the rim of the skin. Bring the opposite sides together to form a semicircle (or triangle if you are using square rather than round won ton skins).

4 Seal by pressing the moistened rim together. Transfer to a cornstarch-dusted plate or cutting board. Cover with a dry kitchen towel.

5 Heat the oil in a nonstick skillet and add as many dumplings as will fill the pan, browning them, about 2 minutes.*

6 Add ½ cup water to the pan and cover immediately. Let steam until the skins are translucent, about 3 minutes.

7 Drain off the water and transfer to a serving dish with a slotted spoon. Serve immediately with Chinese vinegar or soy sauce.

NOTE: Potstickers can be assembled ahead and frozen.

Makes 40 dumplings

* Since the dumplings will not all fit in one pan, you will need to repeat or work with more than one pan.

SPICY YOGURT DIP

1 cup carrots and 2 tablespoons dip provide:
45 calories
74% carbohydrate
13% protein
13% fat
.5 g fat
0.9 mg cholesterol
0.2 g saturated fat
90.0 mg sodium
2.3 g fiber

1 cup nonfat or low-fat plain yogurt

½ cup salsa

1 teaspoon ground cumin

⅛ teaspoon Tabasco sauce

1 Mix all the ingredients well and serve as a dip with vegetables.

Makes 1½ cups

 # QUESADILLA WITH CHEESE AND CILANTRO

3 wedges provide:
59 calories
62% carbohydrate
16% protein
23% fat
1.5 g fat
2 mg cholesterol
0.4 g saturated fat
17 mg sodium
0.3 g fiber

4 flour tortillas

1 ounce part-skim mozzarella cheese, grated

1 zucchini, grated

1 tablespoon chopped cilantro

1 Preheat the oven to 400°. Put 2 tortillas on a baking sheet.

2 Place half the remaining ingredients on 1 tortilla, and half on the other.

3 Top each tortilla with the remaining tortillas to make a pie.

4 Bake for 12 minutes, or until the cheese is melted and the tortillas are slightly crispy.

5 Cut each pie into 6 wedges, and place, in its original shape, on a serving plate. Serve with a dish of salsa in the middle of the pie.

Makes 12 wedges

BAKED TORTILLA CHIPS

1 ounce or 6 Baked Tortilla Chips provide: 67 calories 73% carbohydrate 12% protein 15% fat 1 g fat 0 mg cholesterol 0 g saturated fat 53 mg sodium 1.1 g fiber	12 corn tortillas Seasonings

12 corn tortillas
Seasonings

1 Preheat the oven to 375°. Arrange the tortillas in a stack. Cut the stack in half and then into thirds.
2 Place the wedges on several baking sheets, and season as desired, with garlic, cumin, or cayenne.
3 Bake until the wedges are crisp, about 7 minutes. (Note: Adding a small amount of salt to home-baked chips is still a substantial sodium savings over commercial chips.)

NOTE: The home-baked tortilla chips are thicker than the Doritos. I compare equal weights.

Makes 6 dozen chips

1 ounce (16) Doritos corn chips provide:
155 calories
43% carbohydrate
4% protein
53% fat
9 g fat
0 mg cholesterol
1.5 g saturated fat
164 mg sodium
1.7 g fiber

 # MEXICAN BEAN DIP

½ cup Dip provides:
97 calories
73% carbohydrate
22% protein
5% fat
.5 g fat
0 mg cholesterol
0.1 g saturated fat
598 mg sodium
3 g fiber

1 12-ounce can pinto beans, drained and rinsed
¼ cup canned diced green chilies
1 tablespoon salsa

1 Place all the ingredients in a blender and puree thoroughly.
2 Pour the dip into a saucepan and stir over low heat for 10 minutes.
3 Serve hot or cold with crisped tortilla chips.

Makes 1½ cups

¼ cup refried beans with 1 tablespoon lard provides:
162 calories
21% carbohydrate
7% protein
72% fat
13 g fat
12 mg cholesterol
5 g saturated fat
249 mg sodium
3 g fiber

KITCHEN SINK NACHOS WITH BEAN, CHEESE, AND
 SALSA

60 Baked Tortilla Chips (see recipe on page 236)
1 cup Mexican Bean Dip (see preceding recipe)
8 green chilies, diced
2 ounces mozzarella cheese, grated
¾ cup salsa

1 Preheat the oven to 400°. Spread the chips on several baking sheets.
2 Add the bean dip and chilies to the tortilla chips.
3 Top with the cheese and bake for 5 minutes, or until the cheese is melted.
4 Serve with salsa.

Makes 60 nachos (about 10 servings)

PINEAPPLE SALSA

This salsa was a big hit at one of my Fast-Food Dinner parties. The salsa accompanied a barbecued pork roast as made on my father's farm in Iowa. The pork was served buffet-style along with corn tortillas, black beans, and the Pineapple Salsa.

2 cups fresh pineapple, chopped
1 red bell pepper, chopped (about 1 cup)
½ cup chopped onion (1 small)
1 serrano or jalapeño chili, minced
½ cup chopped fresh coriander or cilantro or 4
   teaspoons dry
Juice of 1 lime
1 tablespoon rice vinegar
Dried crushed red pepper to taste

1 Mix the first 5 ingredients together.
2 Stir in the lime juice, vinegar and red pepper.

(continued on next page)

3 Serve with your favorite grilled fish, chicken, pork, or beef.

Makes 4 cups

NOTE: Substitute papaya for pineapple. Fresh jicama is also a nice addition, if available.

EGGPLANT SLICES WITH MARINARA AND PARMESAN

2 slices of eggplant with homemade sauce provide:
85 calories
52% carbohydrate
14% protein
34% fat
3.5 g fat
3.3 mg cholesterol
1.1 g saturated fat
286 mg sodium
2.1 g fiber

1 large eggplant (approximately 1 pound)
1 cup Marinara Sauce (page 217, or bottled)
¼ cup grated Parmesan cheese

1 Bake whole, unpeeled eggplant in a 350° oven for 35 minutes, or until tender.
2 Remove from the oven, and when cool enough to handle, slice into 1" strips. Place in a shallow baking pan.
3 Top with the sauce and cheese and return to the oven, or microwave until heated through.

VARIATION: Instead of the marinara sauce and cheese, top the slices with a mixture of olive oil, crushed garlic, dried rosemary, and black pepper. Place in a nonstick pan and grill at high heat until slightly brown.

NOTE: See page 217 for comparison of bottled sauce and homemade sauce.

Makes 12 slices

ANTIPASTO WITH VINAIGRETTE

½ cup assorted vegetables with 1 teaspoon Vinaigrette provides:
29 calories
58% carbohydrate
16% protein
25% fat
1 g fat
0 mg cholesterol
0.1 g saturated fat
8.7 mg sodium
1.9 g fiber

3 cups vegetables: broccoli, red onion, carrot, Italian chili peppers, zucchini, cherry tomatoes
1 tablespoon olive oil
1 tablespoon red wine vinegar
2 cloves garlic, crushed
1 teaspoon dried oregano
Salt and pepper to taste

1 Steam the vegetables for 10 minutes. Rinse with cold water.
2 Put them in a bowl.
3 Combine the ingredients for the vinaigrette and drizzle them on the vegetables.
4 Marinate overnight for antipasto.

Makes 6 servings

 # MUSHROOMS IN SHERRY AND TARRAGON

8 mushrooms in sherry provide:
37 calories
41% carbohydrate
17% protein
32% fat
1.5 g fat
0 mg cholesterol
0.2 g saturated fat
8.6 mg sodium
1.5 g fiber

8 fried mushrooms with cheese provide:
166 calories
8% carbohydrate
9% protein
82% fat
16 g fat
4.9 mg cholesterol
3 g saturated fat
118 mg sodium
1.3 g fiber

1 teaspoon olive oil
2 teaspoons tarragon vinegar
¼ teaspoon Dijon mustard
Freshly ground black pepper to taste
2 tablespoons white wine
¾ pound fresh mushrooms (about 32)

1 Place all the ingredients except the mushrooms in a saucepan and bring to a simmer.
2 Add the mushrooms, keeping them whole, and simmer until tender, 3 to 5 minutes.
3 Place in a serving platter, and enjoy.

Makes about 32 mushrooms

ROMAN GRILLED GARLIC TOAST WITH ROMA
 TOMATOES

1 1-ounce slice of toast provides:
131 calories
62% carbohydrate
12% protein
26% fat
3.5 g fat
0 mg cholesterol
0.5 g saturated fat
198 mg sodium
1.6 g fiber

1 loaf sourdough or French bread, sliced in half lengthwise

2 cloves fresh garlic, crushed

3 tablespoons olive oil, or ½ teaspoon per slice of bread

3 Roma tomatoes, sliced (see Note)

1 sprig rosemary, or 1 teaspoon dried

1 Brush the bread halves with the garlic oil.
2 Top with the sliced tomatoes.
3 Place the rosemary over the tomatoes.
4 Grill under a broiler or on an outdoor barbecue until brown.

NOTE: Roma are small, oval tomatoes, but any tomato will do.

Makes 16 slices, depending on size of loaf

CUCUMBER YOGURT DIP

2 tablespoons dip provide:
21 calories
61% carbohydrate
34% protein
4% fat
0 g fat
0.5 mg cholesterol
0 saturated fat
22 mg sodium
0.5 g fiber

1 cup nonfat or low-fat plain yogurt
1 cucumber, chopped
Salt and pepper to taste

Puree the cucumber and yogurt in a food processor or blender and use as a dip for vegetables.

Makes 1 cup

CAJUN PITA TRIANGLES

3 triangles provide:
72 calories
57% carbohydrate
11% protein
32% fat
2.5 g fat
0 mg cholesterol
0.3 g saturated fat
107 mg sodium
0.2 g fiber

Pita bread, one of the recently discovered pleasures from the Middle East, is available everywhere.

2 teaspoons olive oil
2 snack-size pita breads (5" to 6" in diameter)
Cajun seasonings*

1 Brush the oil onto the pita breads and sprinkle with seasonings.
2 Bake in a toaster oven or place under a broiler for 2 minutes, or until lightly browned.
3 Cut each pita into 6 wedges.

Makes 12 triangles

* Cajun seasonings are a blend of spices often containing salt, red pepper, chili peppers, garlic, et cetera, and can generally be found with other seasonings in the supermarket or at the meat or fish counter.

CHAPTER · 16

DESSERTS

People who live fast most likely have a hard enough time cooking a meal, and spending extra time on preparing an elaborate dessert is not likely to happen. Dessert will probably be picked up at a bakery or specialty deli, or, perhaps it is prepared very simply. (If you do opt to prepare a traditional dessert, there are many other wonderful books to turn to. Use the substitution list from Part II, Chapter One to make rich desserts lower in fat and cholesterol.)

Here are some simple ways to end a meal, with 150 calories per serving, rather than 150 calories per mouthful. I am also including a pumpkin pie, because I have so many requests for it around the holidays.

 Grilled Fruit with Sorbet and Mint
Strawberries Dipped in Yogurt and Brown Sugar
Seasonal Berries with Champagne Sauce
Honeydew Melon with Yogurt and Gingersnaps
Pineapple with Yogurt and Fig Bars
Angel Food Cake with Fresh Strawberries
Puree of Frozen Banana
Better Pumpkin Pie

GRILLED FRUIT WITH SORBET AND MINT

Fruit: peaches, apricots, apples, pears, bananas

Narrow-meshed double-grid iron
Brown sugar, honey, cinnamon
Rum or liqueur of choice
Sorbet or lime sherbet
Mint sprigs

PEACHES OR APRICOTS:

1 Cut in half, remove pit.
2 In hollow, place ½ teaspoon honey.

APPLES OR PEARS:

1 Cut in half, cut out core.
2 Score 3 cuts per half in skin, just deep enough to prevent breakage of skin during cooking.
3 Place ½ teaspoon brown sugar in hollowed core of each half.

GRILLING THE FRUIT:

1 Begin with the apples and peaches, placing them in the grid or directly on the barbecue or in a grill rack. Apples and peaches take about 2 minutes longer than other fruit.
2 Add the apricots and pears to the grill.
3 Grill for 7 to 8 minutes on the skin side and for 2 to 3 minutes on the open side, or until slightly charred.
4 Serve on a plate with sorbet and a sprig of mint. Sprinkle with cinnamon, if desired.

NOTE: This is a high-fiber dessert.

STRAWBERRIES DIPPED IN YOGURT AND BROWN SUGAR

½ cup fruit, ½ cup yogurt, and 1 tablespoon brown sugar provide:
137 calories
77% carbohydrate
20% protein
3% fat
.5 g fat
2 mg cholesterol
0.1 g saturated fat
92 mg sodium
1.6 g fiber

1 cup nonfat or low-fat plain yogurt

2 tablespoons brown sugar

1 cup (basket) fresh strawberries, washed

1 Place the strawberries on a platter surrounding a bowl of yogurt and a bowl of brown sugar.

2 Your dining partner will have no problem following your example as you dip the first strawberry in yogurt, then in brown sugar. Fast and elegant.

Makes 2 servings

SEASONAL BERRIES WITH PEACH LIQUEUR SAUCE

½ cup strawberries with 2 tablespoons sauce provides:
127 calories
55% carbohydrate
11% protein
21% fat
3 g fat
137 mg cholesterol
0.9 g saturated fat
36 mg sodium
1.6 g fiber

SAUCE:

2 eggs, separated saving both whites, but only 1 yolk

Pinch salt

2 tablespoons peach schnapps or other flavored liqueur

2 tablespoons sugar

1 cup fresh raspberries or hulled strawberries

1 Beat egg white to stiff peaks

2 In a saucepan whisk the remaining sauce ingredients together for 1 minute.

3 Then add egg whites and whisk over moderately low heat for 3 to 4 minutes, until the sauce becomes thick, foamy, and warm to your finger. Note: Avoid overcooking to result in a "scrambled" eggs consistency.

4 Serve warm or cold over the berries.

NOTE: Analysis done with ½ cup strawberries was 23 calories, .4 g fiber; ½ cup raspberries was 30 calories, 1.8 g fiber (more fiber because of more seeds).

Makes 2 servings

HONEYDEW MELON WITH YOGURT AND
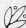 GINGERSNAPS

1 cup honeydew, ¼ cup yogurt, and 2 gingersnaps provide: 160 calories 70% carbohydrate 11% protein 19% fat 3.5 g fat 1 mg cholesterol 0.4 g saturated fat 100 mg sodium 1.5 g fiber

1 cup nonfat plain yogurt

1 honeydew melon, cubed (about 4 cups)

1 lime, halved, reserving 1 slice

8 gingersnaps

1 Place the yogurt in a small bowl and set on a platter.

2 Place the melon chunks around the bowl and squeeze the juice of the lime on the melon. Garnish the yogurt with the slice of lime.

3 Serve with the gingersnaps.

Makes 4 servings

PINEAPPLE WITH YOGURT AND FIG BARS

¼ cup pineapple. (2 rounds), ¼ cup yogurt, and 2 fig bars provide: 176 calories 78% carbohydrates 10% protein 12% fat 2.3 g fat 1 mg cholesterol 0.5 g saturated fat 134 mg sodium 1.2 g fiber

1 pineapple, cut into round slices (save top for garnish, makes about 4 cups)

1 cup nonfat plain yogurt

8 fig bars

1 Place the pineapple top in the center of a platter and surround with the pineapple rounds.

2 Serve with the yogurt and fig bars.

Makes 4 servings

ANGEL FOOD CAKE WITH FRESH STRAWBERRIES

⅟₁₆ of cake provides:
177 calories
89% carbohydrate
10% protein
1% fat
0 g fat
0 mg cholesterol
0 g saturated fat
159 mg sodium
0.8 g fiber

1 cup fresh strawberries
1 large angel food cake (purchased from supermarket bakery)
1 cup all-fruit strawberry jam
3 tablespoons rum (optional)

1 Place the strawberries evenly around the top of the cake.
2 Combine the jam and rum, if desired, in a small saucepan and bring to a boil while stirring.
3 Boil for 3 minutes, or until the jam falls from the spoon in thick drops.
4 Drizzle the hot glaze over the cake and serve.

NOTE: This is a very low-fat dessert—great for birthday cake.

Makes 16 servings

PUREE OF FROZEN BANANA

½ cup provides:
105 calories
92% carbohydrate
4% protein
4% fat
.5 g fat
0 mg cholesterol
0.2 g saturated fat
1 mg sodium
2.7 g fiber

4 ripe bananas, peeled and sliced
1 teaspoon vanilla extract

1 Freeze the banana slices for several hours or overnight.
2 Thaw slightly and puree in a food processor or blender.
3 Add in the vanilla; mix.
4 Pour into 4 dessert dishes and serve.

Makes 4 servings; 2 cups

BETTER PUMPKIN PIE

1½ cups canned pumpkin

¾ cup sugar

½ teaspoon salt

1 teaspoon cinnamon

½–1 teaspoon ground ginger

¼ teaspoon ground cloves

¼ teaspoon ground nutmeg

2 egg yolks

3 egg whites

1¼ cup low-fat milk

1 6-ounce can evaporated skim milk

1 9-inch piecrust (pastry shell)

1 Preheat oven to 425°.

2 Combine pumpkin with dry ingredients.

3 Slightly beat egg yolks with egg whites; then blend with low-fat milk and evaporated skim milk.

4 Pour into pastry shell.

5 Bake for 15 minutes, then lower oven temperature to 300° and bake for 1 hour and 20 minutes or until knife comes out clean.

Makes 8 servings

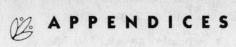

APPENDICES

APPENDIX A:

RATING SYSTEM FORMULATION

+1   30–35% of calories from fat

+2   less than 30% of calories from fat

+1   10–15% saturated fat

+2   less than 10% saturated fat

+1   less than 90 milligrams cholesterol

+1   less than 600 milligrams sodium

+1   greater than or equal to 1.5 grams fiber

+2   greater than or equal to 25% RDA of 4 nutrients (A, C, Iron, Calcium) average for a meal, greater than or equal to 10% of the same nutrients averaged for a single item

+1   greater than or equal to 10–25% RDA of 4 nutrients (A, C, Iron, Calcium) are averaged for a meal, 5–10% of the same nutrients averaged for a single item

+1   less than 5 grams added sugar (1 teaspoon)

Here are a few examples of how foods are rated using the scale in Appendix A, on page 249:

1. McDonald's Big Mac: 560 calories, 32.4 g fat, 10.1 g saturated fat, 103 mg cholesterol, 950 mg sodium, <1.5 g fiber, <5 g sugar, and 50 percent of the combined U.S. RDA for vitamin A, vitamin C, iron, and calcium. First, percentages are calculated for percent of calories from fat and percent of calories from saturated fat. There are 9 calories/g of fat, so a Big Mac gets 52 percent of calories from fat and 17.5 percent of calories from saturated fat. Now, starting with 10, points are subtracted for nutritional factors not meeting the criteria listed above. Therefore, 4 points are lost for the fat and saturated fat content, 1 point is lost for the >90 mg cholesterol, 1 point is lost for the >600 mg sodium, and 1 point is lost for <1.5 g of dietary fiber. The only points that remain are the 2 points for the Big Mac meeting more than 40 percent of the U.S. RDA for the nutrients listed above, and for having <5 g of sugar which gives it a rating of 3.

2. Weight Watchers Chicken Burrito: This item is considered a meal since it is a frozen dinner including a vegetable medley. 310 calories, 13 g fat, 4 g saturated fat, 60 mg cholesterol, 790 mg sodium, <1.5 g dietary fiber, <5 g sugar, and 31 percent of the combined U.S. RDA for the nutrients listed above. The amount of calories from fat is 38 percent and 11.6 percent from saturated fat. Starting from 10, 2 points are subtracted for the fat content, and 1 point for the saturated fat content. One point is lost for >600 mg sodium and 1 for <1.5 g fiber. Two points are subtracted for combined percentage of U.S. RDA less than 40 percent yielding a final rating of 3.

3. 1 oz. (6) Nabisco Triscuit wafers: 120 calories, 4 g fat, <2 g saturated fat, 0 mg cholesterol, 150 mg sodium, <1.5 dietary fiber, <5 g sugar, and <16 percent combined U.S. RDA for the above nutrients. Starting from 10, 1 point is subtracted for 30 percent of calories from fat, saturated fat is less than 10 percent of calories. A point is lost for the fiber content and 2 points are lost for containing less than 20 percent of U.S. RDA combined for the above nutrients. Therefore, the final rating is 6.

APPENDIX B:

CHOLESTEROL AND FAT CONTENT OF COMMON FOODS, ACCORDING TO FOOD GROUPS

	Cholesterol (mg)	Fat (g)
PROTEIN FOODS:		
½ cup boiled lentils	0	0.4
½ cup canned kidney beans	0	0.5
3 oz. fresh cod	33	<1
3 oz. baked sole or flounder	59	1
3 oz. canned tuna, in water	30	1.5
3 oz. raw clams	42	1.4
3 oz. baked light meat chicken, no skin	72	3.8
3 oz. lean roast beef	56	5.9
3 oz. lean cooked lamb	80	8.5
3.5 oz. roasted, cured ham	53	9
2 tbsp. peanut butter	0	16
1 egg	213	5.6
3 oz. canned shrimp	128	0.9
3 oz. cooked ground beef	88	15.6
3 oz. pan-fried beef liver	372	9
DAIRY PRODUCTS:		
1 c. plain, skim yogurt	4	0.4
1 c. skim milk	5	0.6
4 oz. Simple Pleasures frozen dessert	<15	<1
½ c. 1% low-fat cottage cheese	6	2.3
1 c. 1% low-fat milk	10	2.5
1 oz. Light 'n' Lively swiss or cheddar cheese	15	3
1 c. plain low-fat yogurt	14	3.5
1 oz. Kraft Light Naturals reduced-fat cheese	20	4
½ c. 2% cottage cheese	10	4.4
1 oz. part-skim mozzarella cheese	16	4.5
1 c. 2% fat milk	18	5
¼ c. part-skim ricotta cheese	20	5
1 oz. lite cream cheese	15	5
1 oz. mozzarella cheese	22	6.1
1 oz. feta cheese	25	6
1 oz. hard parmesan cheese	19	7.3
1 oz. swiss cheese	26	7.8
1 c. whole milk	34	8
1 oz. American processed cheese	27	8.9
1 oz. cheddar cheese	30	9.4
1 oz. regular cream cheese	28	10
4 oz. vanilla ice cream	50	12

CHOLESTEROL AND FAT CONTENT OF COMMON FOODS, ACCORDING TO FOOD GROUPS

	Cholesterol (mg)	Fat (g)
FRUITS AND VEGETABLES:		
½ c. all dark green vegetables	0	<1
½ c. all citrus fruits, apples, & peaches	0	<.5
½ c. banana & berries	0	<1
1 baked potato	0	<.5
⅓ medium avocado	0	10
20 pieces french fried potatoes	0	20
GRAIN PRODUCTS:		
½ c. pasta or rice	0	<1
1 slice white or wheat bread	0	1
1/12 angel food cake	0	0
4 whole-grain rye wafers	0	0.4
3 c. plain popcorn	0	0.9
10 saltines	0	3
1 croissant	4	10
COMBINATION FOODS:		
peanut butter & jelly sandwich (as specified in book)	0	11.5
turkey sandwich (as specified in book)	65	5
2 slices Pizza Hut Cheese Pan Pizza	34	18
McDonald's Hamburger	37	9.5
Healthy Choice chicken and vegetables	35	1
Light & Elegant beef stroganoff	65	6
¾ c. Kraft Macaroni & Cheese	5	13

NOTE: CHOLESTEROL OCCURS ONLY IN FOODS OF ANIMAL ORIGIN.

APPENDIX C:

FIBER CONTENT OF COMMON FOODS

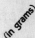

Food	(in grams)
1 c. cooked black-eyed peas	24.8
½ c. baked beans	11.0
1 c. cooked green peas	10.7
1 c. cooked lima beans	8.7
1 c. boiled lentils	7.9
1 c. cooked black beans	7.2
1 c. cooked brussel sprouts	7.2
1 c. boiled kidney beans	6.4
1 c. boiled chickpeas	5.7
1 c. chili w/beans	5.1
1 baked potato w/skin	4.9
1 c. cooked green beans	4.6
1 c. cooked onions	4.4
1 medium pear	4.1
1 c. cooked spinach	4.0
1 c. canned mixed vegetables	3.9
1 orange	3.6
1 ear cooked corn	3.6
1 c. grated carrots	3.6
1 c. mashed potatoes	3.4
1 c. strawberries	3.2
1 medium apple w/skin	2.8
½ cantaloupe	2.7
10 potato chips	2.4
1 c. pineapple pieces	2.4
½ medium avocado	2.4
1 baked sweet potato	2.1
1 c. raw mushrooms	1.8
1 slice whole wheat bread	1.6
1 medium banana	1.6
1 c. spaghetti	1.5
1 tbsp. peanut butter	1.1
1 corn tortilla	1.0
1 stalk celery	0.9
1 water bagel	0.6
1 slice white or sourdough bread	0.1

APPENDIX D:

SODIUM CONTENT OF COMMON FOODS

Food	(in mg)
1 tsp. salt	2130
1 tbsp. soy sauce	825
1 c. beef bouillon	782
1 tbsp. teriyaki sauce	690
6 oz. V-8 juice	593
1 oz. hard Parmesan cheese	454
1 large pancake	431
1 oz. American cheese	406
1 English muffin	364
1 strip bacon	360
1 oz. feta cheese	316
1 oz. pickle relish	300
1 c. corn flakes cereal	300
1 c. buttermilk	257
¼ c. 1% fat cottage cheese	230
¼ c. 2% fat cottage cheese	230
1 tbsp. tartar sauce	220
¼ c. whole cottage cheese	213
1 bagel	198
1 tbsp. mustard	195
¼ c. Grape-nuts cereal	188
1 oz. cheddar cheese	176
1 oz. lite cream cheese	160
1 slice whole wheat bread	159
1 tbsp. ketchup	156
1 c. hot cocoa	140
1 oz. part-skim mozzarella cheese	132
1 tbsp. barbeque sauce	127
1 c. skim milk	126
1 tbsp. butter	123
1 slice white bread	123
1 c. 1% fat milk	123
1 c. 2% fat milk	122
1 c. whole milk	122
1 tbsp. margarine	110
1 oz. mozzarella cheese	106
1 oz. regular cream cheese	86
1 tbsp. mayonnaise	80
2 saltine crackers	80
1 oz. Swiss cheese	74
10 dried apple rings	56
1 corn tortilla	53
1 c. club soda	50

SODIUM CONTENT OF COMMON FOODS

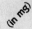

(in mg)

1 c. lemon-lime soda	27
1 c. cantaloupe	14
10 dried peach halves	9
1 c. cola	9
1 c. Kool-aid	8
½ c. canned fruit cocktail in syrup	7
1 c. diet soda	7
1 c. tea	7
1 c. coffee	6
1 c. fruit juice	5
4 raw apricots	4
½ c. canned fruit cocktail in juice	4
1 c. cooked pasta noodles	3
10 dried apricot halves	3
1 c. raw strawberries	2
⅔ c. cooked oatmeal	1
1 apple	1
½ c. frozen strawberries	1
1 banana	1
1 orange	1
1 c. shredded wheat cereal	<1
1 raw peach	0
1 c. raw raspberries	0
½ c. frozen raspberries	0
½ grapefruit	0

INDEX

juice and juice drinks, 27, 74, 82

Kentucky Fried Chicken, 143
kidney beans:
    chili (soup), **198**
    and garbanzo beans with cauliflower, **191–192**
Kid's Cuisine, 62
kitchen sink nachos with bean, cheese, and salsa, **237**

labels, 17, 70, 71
lamb shish kabob with cherry tomatoes and peppers, **204–5**
late-night snacking, 69–70
leftovers, 45, 61, 168–69
lentil soup, **200**
lifestyle, 84–85, 113–15
lime cream sauce, fettucine with mushrooms, bell peppers, and peas in, **220–21**
linguini:
    with clam sauce, **218–19**
    with shrimp and broccoli, **222**
Long John Silver's, 143–45
lox, cream cheese, and bagel, **181**
lunches, 25, 39–53, 64
    calorie intake at, 39–41
    cheese at, 45–46, 50
    at delis, 42–44
    eaten at home, 51
    Fast-Food Rating Scale for, 42–49, 52–53
    at fast-food restaurants, 40–42
    importance of, 39
    at restaurants, 45, 46–49
    rules for, 39–40
    sandwiches at, 42–43, 45, 49–51, 52
    skipping, 84
    at workplace cafeterias, 44–45
    see also brown-bag lunches

main dishes, **201–31**
    baked swordfish steaks with lemon, tomato, and cracked peppercorns, **213**
    barbecued chicken breasts with Tabasco and lime, **209**
    barbecued (or charred) teriyaki flank steak, **204**
    blackened halibut, **214**
    Cajun chicken, **210**
    chicken enchiladas with lettuce and tomatoes, **211**
    chicken Parmesan with pasta, **212–13**
    chicken pot roast with rosemary and garlic, **210**
    coq au vin, **212**
    Cuban-style beef in tortilla, **225**
    fajitas with chicken and bell peppers, **224**
    fish taco with cabbage, **226**
    fresh tomato pizza, **207–8**
    fried rice with zucchini and mushrooms, **222**
    mozzarella and tomato pizza with spinach, **208–9**
    pan-sautéed snapper with mushrooms and bell peppers, **214**
    rice and peas with water chestnuts, **223**
    roasted turkey breast, **205**
    rosemary chicken with artichoke hearts, **211**
    Santa Fe skewers with shrimp, **216**
    scallops in wine with tomato, **216**
    shish kabob with lamb, cherry tomatoes, and peppers, **204–5**
    shrimp with garlic, **215**
    shrimp with snow peas, **215**
    Spanish fried rice, **223**
    turkey burgers, **206**
    turkey loaf with carrots, **206–7**
    see also pasta; vegetarian main dishes
marinades:
    ginger, **233**
    for shrimp, **216**
marinara sauce:
    eggplant slices with Parmesan and, **238**
    spaghetti squash with, **231**
    spaghetti with, **217**
marinated cucumber slices, **189**
mashed potatoes with cabbage, **227**
mayonnaise, 50, 51
McDonald's, 32, 41, 85, 129–30, 131, 132, 133, 134, 145–46